Other Best-selling Books

OBSTETRICS NURSING PROCEDURE MANUAL

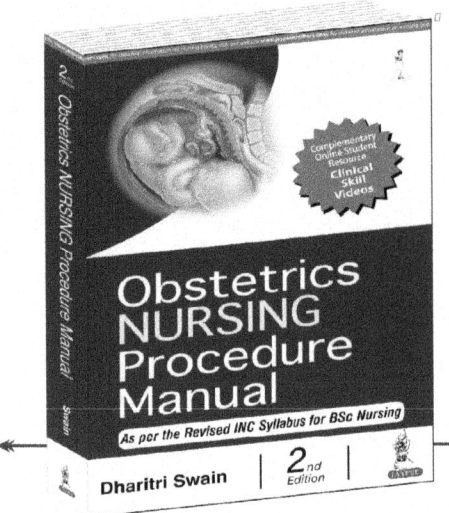

Dharitri Swain
Two Color | Soft Cover | 2/e, 2023
6.75" x 9.5" | 468 Pages | 9789354658938

PEDIATRIC NURSING (FREE! PEDIATRIC NURSING PROCEDURES VIDEOS)

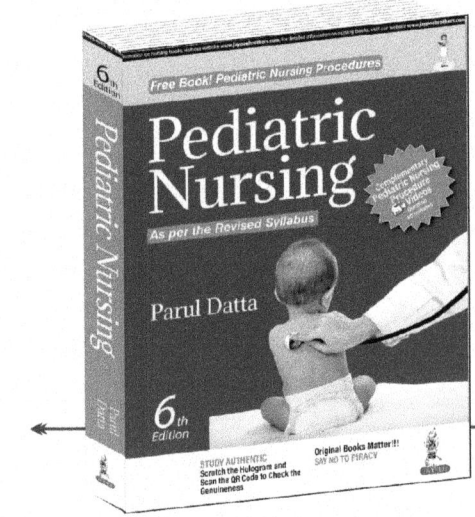

Parul Datta
Two Color | Soft Cover | 6/e, 2023
8.5" x 11" | 544 Pages | 9789356962354

JAYPEE
The Health Sciences Publisher

Please visit our website
www.jaypeebrothers.com or Scan the QR Code

Practical Book for Mental Health Nursing–II
For BSc Nursing Students

Name of the Student _____

Roll Number _____

Name of the Institute _____

Practical Book for Mental Health Nursing–II
For BSc Nursing Students

As per the Revised Nursing Syllabus

SECOND EDITION

Bushra Mushtaq PG (Psychiatric Nursing)
Tutor (AMMCN and MT)
Islamic University of Science and Technology
Awantipora, Jammu and Kashmir, India

Javaid Ahmad Mir PG (Psychiatric Nursing)
Faculty, Government Nursing College
GMC, Baramulla, Jammu and Kashmir, India

Foreword
Mohammad Ayoub Dar

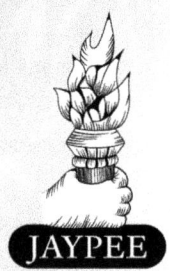

JAYPEE BROTHERS MEDICAL PUBLISHERS
The Health Sciences Publisher
New Delhi | London

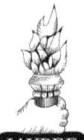 **Jaypee Brothers Medical Publishers (P) Ltd**

Headquarters
Jaypee Brothers Medical Publishers (P) Ltd
EMCA House, 23/23-B
Ansari Road, Daryaganj
New Delhi 110 002, India
Landline: +91-11-23272143, +91-11-23272703
+91-11-23282021, +91-11-23245672
Email: jaypee@jaypeebrothers.com

Overseas Office
J.P. Medical Ltd
83 Victoria Street, London
SW1H 0HW (UK)
Phone: +44 20 3170 8910
Email: info@jpmedpub.com

Corporate Office
Jaypee Brothers Medical Publishers (P) Ltd
4838/24, Ansari Road, Daryaganj
New Delhi 110 002, India
Phone: +91-11-43574357
Fax: +91-11-43574314
Email: jaypee@jaypeebrothers.com

EU GPSR Authorised Representative
Logos Europe, 9 rue Nicolas Poussin
17000, La Rochelle, France
Phone: +33 (0) 6 67 93 73 78
E-mail: Contact@logoseurope.eu

Website: www.jaypeebrothers.com
Website: www.jaypeedigital.com

© 2024, Jaypee Brothers Medical Publishers

The views and opinions expressed in this book are solely those of the original contributor(s)/author(s) and do not necessarily represent those of editor(s) and publisher of the book.

All rights reserved. No part of this publication may be reproduced, stored or transmitted in any form or by any means, electronic, mechanical, photocopying, recording or otherwise, without the prior permission in writing of the publishers.

All brand names and product names used in this book are trade names, service marks, trademarks or registered trademarks of their respective owners. The publisher is not associated with any product or vendor mentioned in this book.

Medical knowledge and practice change constantly. This book is designed to provide accurate, authoritative information about the subject matter in question. However, readers are advised to check the most current information available on procedures included and check information from the manufacturer of each product to be administered, to verify the recommended dose, formula, method and duration of administration, adverse effects and contraindications. It is the responsibility of the practitioner to take all appropriate safety precautions. Neither the publisher nor the author(s)/editor(s) assume any liability for any injury and/or damage to persons or property arising from or related to use of material in this book.

This book is sold on the understanding that the publisher is not engaged in providing professional medical services. If such advice or services are required, the services of a competent medical professional should be sought.

Every effort has been made where necessary to contact holders of copyright to obtain permission to reproduce copyright material. If any have been inadvertently overlooked, the publisher will be pleased to make the necessary arrangements at the first opportunity.

Inquiries for bulk sales may be solicited at: jaypee@jaypeebrothers.com

Practical Book for Mental Health Nursing–II

First Edition: 2022
Second Edition: **2024**
ISBN: 978-93-5696-833-2

FOREWORD

I am delighted to offer my insights for inclusion in the *Practical Book for Mental Health Nursing-II*. Mental health nursing is a discipline that demands a nuanced understanding of the complexities of the human mind, coupled with the compassionate care that defines the nursing profession.

In this comprehensive practical book, students will find a valuable resource that transcends theoretical concepts and delves into the practicalities of mental health nursing. The crucial juncture where theoretical knowledge begins to take tangible shape in clinical practice. This practical book serves as a guide, providing a bridge between classroom learning and the dynamic challenges of mental health care.

Authored by dedicated professionals with extensive experience in mental health nursing, this practical book incorporates real-world scenarios, case studies, and practical exercises that mirror the complexities faced in clinical settings. It encourages active engagement, critical thinking, and the development of essential skills required for effective mental health nursing practice.

As the field of mental health nursing evolves, so do the challenges and opportunities it presents. This practical book equips students not only with foundational knowledge but also with the adaptability and resilience needed to navigate the ever-changing landscape of mental health care.

I commend the authors for their commitment to advancing mental health nursing education and providing students with a valuable tool for their academic and professional journey. I believe that this practical book will be an asset to students, educators, and practitioners alike, fostering a culture of excellence and compassion in mental health nursing.

I extend my best wishes to the students who embark on the exploration of mental health nursing through this practical book. May it inspire you, challenge you, and ultimately empower you to make meaningful contributions to the well-being of those in your care.

Warm regards,

Mohammad Ayoub Dar
Assistant Professor
Mader-E-Meharban Institute of Nursing
Sciences and Research SKIMS
Srinagar, Jammu and Kashmir, India

PREFACE TO THE SECOND EDITION

It is our distinct privilege to present second edition of *Practical Book for Mental Health Nursing–II*, a resource tailored to meet the evolving needs of nursing students entering the crucial phase of their mental health education. This practical book aims to serve as a dynamic companion, offering a blend of theoretical foundations and practical applications essential for navigating the intricate landscape of mental health care. Drawing upon my experience and commitment to advancing nursing education, practical book is designed to empower nursing students with the knowledge, skills, and critical thinking abilities necessary for delivering compassionate and evidence-based care. We trust that this comprehensive practical book will not only enhance academic learning but also instill confidence in students as they embark on their clinical journey in mental health nursing.

Javaid Ahmad Mir
Bushra Mushtaq

PREFACE TO THE FIRST EDITION

Welcome to the first edition of *Practical Book for Mental Health Nursing*.

This practical book is designed to help students to perform effectively and efficiently in clinical settings. The goal of this practical book is to provide the students tools for record keeping in nursing profession. The contents and procedures are designed for clinical purposes only.

This practical book is user-friendly and cost-effective for students as the contents in this book are so arranged that it covers entire clinical experience for nursing students and make easy for evaluators and instructors to evaluate the students performance at one platform. We are welcome any comments or suggestions for this record book; it will make the next edition better.

Bushra Mushtaq
Javaid Ahmad Mir

ACKNOWLEDGMENTS

On the recollection of so many great blessings, I now, with a high sense of gratitude, presume to offer my sincere thanks to the Almighty, the Creator and the Preserver. No deed can find the reality without the grace of Almighty. I would like to express deepest sense of everlasting gratitude to the "Almighty Allah" for giving me strength and showered his marvellous blessings during the whole study.

We express our profound respect and deep gratitude to our parents **Mr and Mrs GA Mir** and **Mr and Mrs Mushtaq Ahmad Bhat,** for their support, valuable suggestions and guidance.

We evince our admiration and special thanks of gratitude to **Ms Parkash Kour, and Mr Ayoub Dar** precious opinion and unremitting support which made our work smooth and successful.

We extend our heartfelt gratitude and appreciation to all our **teachers** for the invaluable gift of knowledge and guidance you have shared with us. Your unwavering dedication to teaching has not only enriched our minds but also inspired us to strive for excellence.

We want to extend our sincere gratitude to each one of you for your valuable comments and feedback on the last edition of our publication. Your insights and suggestions have played a pivotal role in shaping the improved quality and content of this current edition.

This project would never have taken the shape without support and help from, **Mr Rameez Jogi (The Nurses' crib).**

We are thankful to our siblings and their partners for their tremendous support in helping and supporting this project. We are thankful to our **brother Er. Faisal Ahmad Mir and sisters Ms Shaheena, Adv. Sameena Anjum, Ms Onaisa Aalia Mushtaq , Ms Mohsina Aalia Mushtaq** for their valuable suggestions especially.

We express our humble thanks to Shri Jitendar P Vij (Group Chairman), Mr Ankit Vij (Managing Director), Mr MS Mani (Group President), Dr Madhu Choudhary (Director-Educational Publishing), Ms Pooja Bhandari [Director-Production (Books and Journals)], Ms Sunita Katla (Executive Assistant to Group Chairman and Publishing Manager), Mr Ajay Kumar Sharma [Deputy General Manager (Books and Journals)], Ms Samina Khan (Executive Assistant to Director-Educational Publishing), Ms Jitika Royal (Content Strategist-Nursing), Mr Rajesh Sharma (Production Coordinator), Ms Seema Dogra (Cover Visualizer), Mr Rahul Jadli (Proofreader), Mr Om Prakash Mishra (Typesetter), Mr Sharvan Kumar (Graphic Designer) of M/S Jaypee Brothers Medical Publishers (P) Ltd, New Delhi, India an exclusive medical books publishing house for publishing this project.

We dedicate this book to our twin daughters **Mafaz Javaid and Manal Javaid.**

CERTIFICATE OF CLINICAL EXPERIENCE

Student's Name: _____

Class Roll No.: _____

Examination Roll No.: _____

College/Institute: _____

Paste a recent passport size photograph.

Student's Declaration:

I _____ CERTIFY that I have completed the Psychiatric Clinical Posting for 6th semester nursing program and gained professional experience, knowledge and skills under supervision as detailed in my procedure book. All the contents in my procedure record book are true and real to the best of my knowledge.

Places of posting:

1. Name of Hospital: _____
   Address: _____
2. Name of Hospital: _____
   Address: _____
3. Name of Hospital: _____
   Address: _____

Student's Signature

_____

Instructor's Declaration:

I CERTIFY that this student has completed the Psychiatric Clinical Posting for 6th semester nursing program in accordance with the guidelines provided by institution and has, in my opinion, reached a level of professional experience expected from a 6th semester student.

Instructor's Signature　　　　　　　　　　　　　　　　　　　　　　　**Principal's Signature**

_____　　　　　　　　　　　　　　　　　　　　　　_____

Internal Examiner's Signature　　　　　　　　　　　　　　　　　　**External Examiner's Signature**

_____　　　　　　　　　　　　　　　　　　　　　　_____

Date____/_____/_____　　　　　　　　　　　　　　　　　　　　Date____/_____/_____

PEDAGOGY

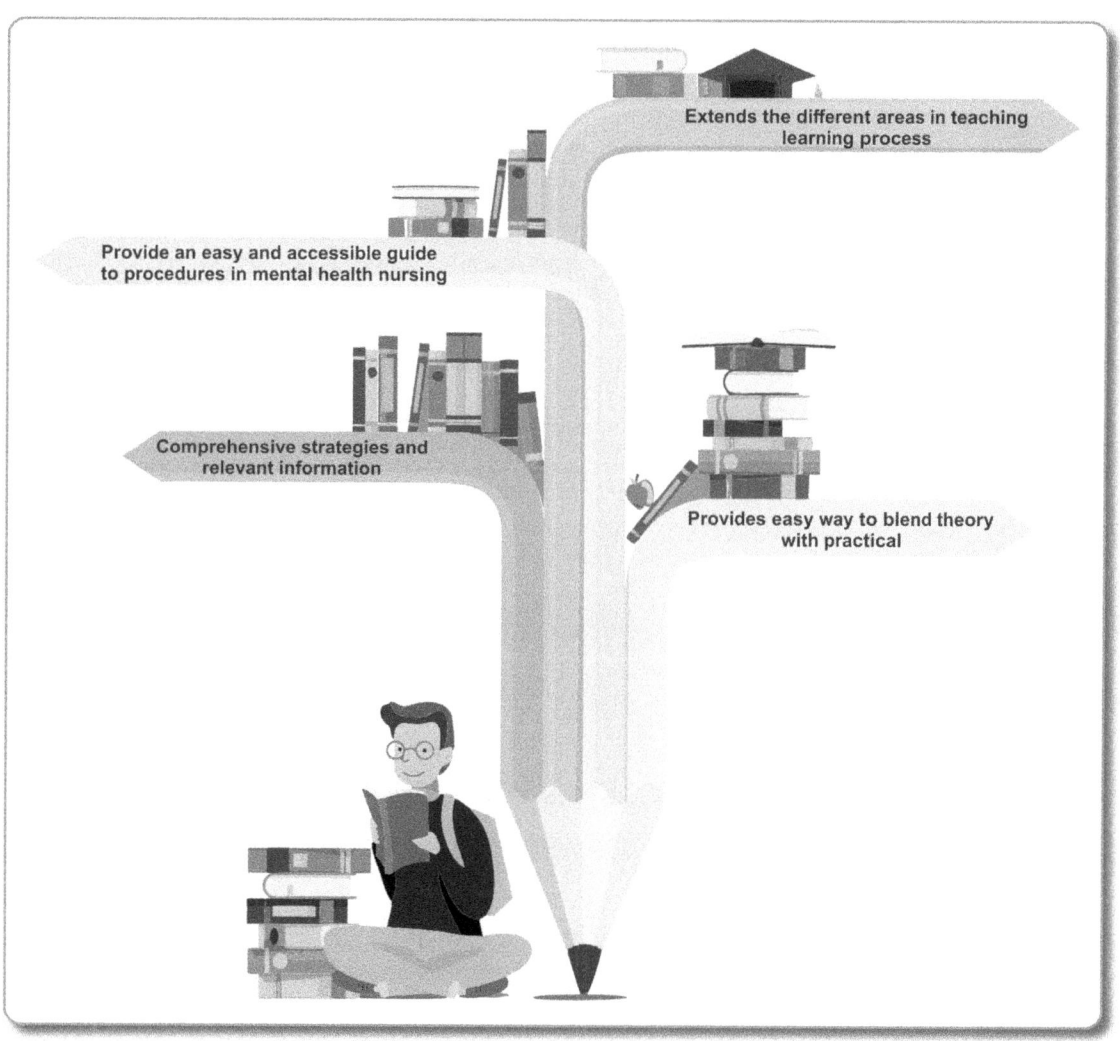

CONTENTS

1.	History Taking	1
2.	Physical Assessment	19
3.	Mental Status Examination (MSE)	37
4.	Mini-Mental Status Examination (MMSE)	65
5.	Neurological Examination	73
6.	Process Recording	101
7.	ECT (Electroconvulsive Therapy)	119
8.	Therapies	131
9.	Psychometric Assessment	139
10.	Case Study	147
11.	Community Mental Health Nursing: Case Work	197
12.	Community Mental Health Nursing: Individual Care Plan	217
13.	Community Mental Health Nursing: Family Care Plan	223
14.	Drug Book	231
14.	Health Education	239
16.	Mental Health Camp	243

SYLLABUS

CLINICAL PRACTICUM
MENTAL HEALTH NURSING – I AND II

PLACEMENT: Semester V and VI
MENTAL HEALTH NURSING – I: 1 credit (80 hours)
MENTAL HEALTH NURSING – II: 2 credits (160 hours)
Practice competencies: On completion of the course, the students will be able to:
1. Assess patients with mental health problems/disorders.
2. Observe and assist in various treatment modalities or therapies.
3. Counsel and educate patients and families.
4. Perform individual and group psychoeducation.
5. Provide nursing care to patients with mental health problems/disorders.
6. Motivate patients in the community for early treatment and follow up.
7. Observe the assessment and care of patients with substance abuse disorders in deaddiction center.

CLINICAL POSTINGS
(8 weeks × 30 hours per week = 240 hours)

Clinical area/ unit	Duration (weeks)	Learning outcomes	Skills/procedural competencies	Clinical requirements	Assessments methods
Psychiatric OPD	2	• Assess patients with mental health problems • Observe and assist in therapies • Counsel and educate patients, and families	• History taking • Perform mental status examination (MSE) • Observe/practice psychometric assessment • Perform neurological examination • Observing and assisting in therapies • Individual and group psycho- education • Mental hygiene practice education • Family psychoeducation	• History taking and mental status examination – 2 • Health education – 1 • Observation report of OPD	• Assess performance with rating scale • Assess each skill with checklist • Evaluation of health education • Assessment of observation report • Completion of activity record
Child guidance clinic	1	• Assess children with various mental health problems • Counsel and educate children, families and significant others	• History and mental status examination • Observe/practice psychometric assessment • Observe and assist in various therapies • Parental teaching for child with mental deficiency	• Case work – 1 • Observation report of different therapies – 1	• Assess performance with rating scale • Assess each skill with checklist • Evaluation of the observation report

Clinical area/ unit	Duration (weeks)	Learning outcomes	Skills/procedural competencies	Clinical requirements	Assessments methods
Inpatient ward	4	• Assess patients with mental health problems • Provide nursing care for patients with various mental health problems • Assist in various therapies • Counsel and educate patients, families and significant others	• History taking • Mental status examination (MSE) • Neurological examination • Assisting in psychometric assessment • Recording therapeutic communication • Administration of medications • Assist electroconvulsive therapy (ECT) • Participating in all therapies • Preparing patients for activities of daily living (ADL) • Conducting admission and discharge counseling • Counseling and teaching patients and families	• Give care to 2–3 patients with various mental disorders • Case study – 1 • Care plan • Clinical presentation – 1 • Process recording – 2 • Maintain drug book	• Assess performance with rating scale • Assess each skill with checklist • Evaluation of the case study, care plan, clinical presentation, process recording • Completion of activity record
Community psychiatry and deaddiction center	1	• Identify patients with various mental disorders • Motivate patients for early treatment and follow up • Assist in follow up clinic • Counsel and educate patient, family and community • Observe the assessment and care of patients at deaddiction center	• Conduct home visit and case work • Identifying individuals with mental health problems • Assisting in organizations of Mental Health Camp • Conducting awareness meetings for mental health and mental illness • Counseling and teaching family members, patients and community • Observing deaddiction care	• Case work – 1 • Observation report on field visits • Visit to deaddiction center	• Assess performance with rating scale • Evaluation of case work and observation report • Completion of activity record

HISTORY TAKING

History Taking: Psychiatric history involves the patient's mental outline that includes information about the chief complaint, present illness, medical and surgical records family and individual history, psychological deviation from the onset of the disease and history of childhood development, habits, etc., this history detail of patient should give a comprehensive details of disease.

History Taking – 1

A. Identification Data

Name:	
Age:	
Gender:	
Address:	
Education:	
Occupation:	
Marital status:	
Religion:	
Informant:	

B. Presenting Chief Complaints

_____

_____

_____

C. History of Present Illness

Duration:	
Mode of onset:	
Course:	
Intensity:	

- **Predisposing factor:**

- **Precipitating factor:**

- **Perpetuating factor:**

D. Treatment History

_____

_____

E. Past Psychiatric and Medical History

_____

_____

F. Family History

_____

_____

Age	Education	Occupation	Health status	Relationship with patient	Age at death	Mode of death

Family Tree

G. Personal History

a. Prenatal history: _____

b. Childhood history: _____

Primary caregiver:	
Feeding:	
Developmental milestones:	
Behavioral and emotional problems:	
Illness during childhood:	

c. Educational history: _____

d. Play history: _____

e. Emotional problems during adolescence: _____

f. Puberty: _____

g. Occupational history: _____

h. Sexual and marital history: _____

i. Menstrual and obstetric history (in case of female patient): _____

j. Forensic history: _____

k. Substance abuse history: _____

l. Pre-morbid personality:

Interpersonal relationships:	
Family and social relationships:	
Use of leisure time:	
Habits:	
Eating pattern:	
Predominant mood:	
Religious beliefs:	
Eating pattern:	
Elimination:	
Sleep:	

Signature of Student Nurse   **Signature of Supervisor**

History Taking – 2

A. Identification Data

Name:	
Age:	
Gender:	
Address:	
Education:	
Occupation:	
Marital status:	
Religion:	
Informant:	

B. Presenting Chief Complaints

___

___

C. History of Present Illness

Duration:	
Mode of onset:	
Course:	
Intensity:	

- Predisposing factor:

- Precipitating factor:

- Perpetuating factor:

D. Treatment History

___

___

E. Past Psychiatric and Medical History

_____
_____

F. Family History

_____
_____

Age	Education	Occupation	Health status	Relationship with patient	Age at death	Mode of death

Family Tree

G. Personal History

a. **Prenatal history:** _____
_____
_____

b. **Childhood history:** _____
_____
_____

Primary caregiver:	
Feeding:	
Developmental milestones:	
Behavioral and emotional problems:	
Illness during childhood:	

c. **Educational history:** _____

d. **Play history:** _____

e. **Emotional problems during adolescence:** _____

f. **Puberty:** _____

g. **Occupational history:** _____

h. **Sexual and marital history:** _____

i. **Menstrual and obstetric history (in case of female patient):** _____

j. **Forensic history:** _____

k. **Substance abuse history:** _____

l. **Pre-morbid personality:**

Interpersonal relationships:	
Family and social relationships:	
Use of leisure time:	
Habits:	
Eating pattern:	
Predominant mood:	
Religious beliefs:	
Eating pattern:	
Elimination:	
Sleep:	

Signature of Student Nurse   **Signature of Supervisor**

History Taking – 3

A. Identification Data

Name:	
Age:	
Gender:	
Address:	
Education:	
Occupation:	
Marital status:	
Religion:	
Informant:	

B. Presenting Chief Complaints

___

C. History of Present Illness

Duration:	
Mode of onset:	
Course:	
Intensity:	

- **Predisposing factor:**

- **Precipitating factor:**

- **Perpetuating factor:**

D. Treatment History

___

E. Past Psychiatric and Medical History

_____

_____

F. Family History

_____

_____

Age	Education	Occupation	Health status	Relationship with patient	Age at death	Mode of death

Family Tree

G. Personal History

a. **Prenatal history:** _____

b. **Childhood history:** _____

Primary caregiver:	
Feeding:	
Developmental milestones:	
Behavioral and emotional problems:	
Illness during childhood:	

c. **Educational history:** _____

d. **Play history:** _____

e. **Emotional problems during adolescence:** _____

f. **Puberty:** _____

g. **Occupational history:** _____

h. **Sexual and marital history:** _____

i. **Menstrual and obstetric history (in case of female patient):** _____

j. **Forensic history:** _____

k. **Substance abuse history:** _____

l. **Pre-morbid personality:**

Interpersonal relationships:	
Family and social relationships:	
Use of leisure time:	
Habits:	
Eating pattern:	
Predominant mood:	
Religious beliefs:	
Eating pattern:	
Elimination:	
Sleep:	

Signature of Student Nurse   **Signature of Supervisor**

History Taking – 4

A. Identification Data

Name:	
Age:	
Gender:	
Address:	
Education:	
Occupation:	
Marital status:	
Religion:	
Informant:	

B. Presenting Chief Complaints

___

___

C. History of Present Illness

Duration:	
Mode of onset:	
Course:	
Intensity:	

- **Predisposing factor:**

- **Precipitating factor:**

- **Perpetuating factor:**

D. Treatment History

___

___

E. Past Psychiatric and Medical History

_____
_____

F. Family History

_____
_____

Age	Education	Occupation	Health status	Relationship with patient	Age at death	Mode of death

Family Tree

G. Personal History

a. **Prenatal history:** _____
   _____
   _____

b. **Childhood history:** _____
   _____
   _____

Primary caregiver:	
Feeding:	
Developmental milestones:	
Behavioral and emotional problems:	
Illness during childhood:	

c. **Educational history:** _____

d. **Play history:** _____

e. **Emotional problems during adolescence:** _____

f. **Puberty:** _____

g. **Occupational history:** _____

h. **Sexual and marital history:** _____

i. **Menstrual and obstetric history (in case of female patient):** ___

j. **Forensic history:** _____

k. **Substance abuse history:** _____

l. **Pre-morbid personality:**

Interpersonal relationships:	
Family and social relationships:	
Use of leisure time:	
Habits:	
Eating pattern:	
Predominant mood:	
Religious beliefs:	
Eating pattern:	
Elimination:	
Sleep:	

Signature of Student Nurse   **Signature of Supervisor**

History Taking – 5

A. Identification Data

Name:	
Age:	
Gender:	
Address:	
Education:	
Occupation:	
Marital status:	
Religion:	
Informant:	

B. Presenting Chief Complaints

C. History of Present Illness

Duration:	
Mode of onset:	
Course:	
Intensity:	

- **Predisposing factor:**

- **Precipitating factor:**

- **Perpetuating factor:**

D. Treatment History

E. Past Psychiatric and Medical History

_____

_____

F. Family History

_____

_____

Age	Education	Occupation	Health status	Relationship with patient	Age at death	Mode of death

Family Tree

History Taking

G. Personal History

a. **Prenatal history:** _____

b. **Childhood history:** _____

Primary caregiver:	
Feeding:	
Developmental milestones:	
Behavioral and emotional problems:	
Illness during childhood:	

c. **Educational history:** _____

d. **Play history:** _____

e. **Emotional problems during adolescence:** _____

f. **Puberty:** _____

g. **Occupational history:** _____

h. **Sexual and marital history:** _____

i. **Menstrual and obstetric history (in case of female patient):** _____

j. **Forensic history:** _____

k. **Substance abuse history:** _____

l. **Pre-morbid personality:**

Interpersonal relationships:	
Family and social relationships:	
Use of leisure time:	
Habits:	
Eating pattern:	
Predominant mood:	
Religious beliefs:	
Eating pattern:	
Elimination:	
Sleep:	

Signature of Student Nurse   **Signature of Supervisor**

PHYSICAL ASSESSMENT

Physical Examination: A detailed general physical examination and systemic examination is important in every case as we need to rule out the organic cause first. The examination includes the general physical examination (weight, height, built, any skin lesions, trauma or burn marks, needle marks, skin tattooing or track marks, pallor, icterus, clubbing, edema, nodes, swelling) followed by systemic examination (CVS, respiratory, and abdominal examination). A brief neurological examination comprising of higher mental functions and cranial nerve examinations, examination of motor and sensory system should be done.

Physical Assessment – 1
Demographic Data

Name:	
Age:	
Gender:	
Address:	
Religion:	
Education:	
Occupation:	
Marital status:	
Informant:	
Date of admission:	
MRD No.:	
Diagnosis:	

Physical Assessment

Vital signs	
Temperature:	
Pulse rate:	
Respiratory rate:	
Blood pressure:	
General appearances	
Height = ft. inches, Weight = kg.	
Head	
Shape, scalp	
Hair	
Color, texture	
Eyes	
Eye brows:	
Eyelashes:	
Eyelids:	
Eyeballs:	
Conjunctiva:	
Pupil:	
Lens:	
Vision:	

Ears	
External ears:	
Hearing:	
Any other observations:	
Nose	
External nares:	
Nostrils:	
Any other observations:	
Mouth	
Lips:	
Tongue:	
Gums:	
Teeth:	
Neck	
Range of motion (ROM):	
Thyroid:	
Lymph nodes:	
Skin	
Color, tone	
Any other observations:	
Upper extremities	
Left arm/hand:	
Right arm/hand:	
Lower extremities	
Left leg/feet:	
Right leg/feet:	
Cardiovascular system	
Heart sounds (Inspection, Palpation, Percussion, Auscultation):	
Respiratory system	
Respiratory sounds (Inspection, Palpation, Percussion, Auscultation):	
Gastrointestinal system	
Appetite:	
Bowel habits:	
Abdominal finding (Inspection, Palpation, Percussion, Auscultation):	

Physical Assessment

Genitourinary system	
Musculoskeletal system	
Gait:	
Posture:	
Central nervous system	
Orientation to • Time: • Place: • Person:	
Speech, e.g., stammering, etc.	

Any other observations during physical examination:

_____

_____

_____

_____

Signature of Student Nurse   **Signature of Supervisor**

Physical Assessment – 2

Demographic Data

Name:	
Age:	
Gender:	
Address:	
Religion:	
Education:	
Occupation:	
Marital status:	
Informant:	
Date of admission:	
MRD No.:	
Diagnosis:	

Physical Assessment

Vital signs	
Temperature:	
Pulse rate:	
Respiratory rate:	
Blood pressure:	
General appearances	
Height = ft. inches, Weight = kg.	
Head	
Shape, scalp	
Hair	
Color, texture	
Eyes	
Eye brows:	
Eyelashes:	
Eyelids:	
Eyeballs:	
Conjunctiva:	
Pupil:	
Lens:	
Vision:	

Ears

External ears:	
Hearing:	
Any other observations:	

Nose

External nares:	
Nostrils:	
Any other observations:	

Mouth

Lips:	
Tongue:	
Gums:	
Teeth:	

Neck

Range of motion (ROM):	
Thyroid:	
Lymph nodes:	

Skin

Color, tone	
Any other observations:	

Upper extremities

Left arm/hand:	
Right arm/hand:	

Lower extremities

Left leg/feet:	
Right leg/feet:	

Cardiovascular system

Heart sounds (Inspection, Palpation, Percussion, Auscultation):	

Respiratory system

Respiratory sounds (Inspection, Palpation, Percussion, Auscultation):	

Gastrointestinal system

Appetite:	
Bowel habits:	
Abdominal finding (Inspection, Palpation, Percussion, Auscultation):	

Genitourinary system	

Musculoskeletal system	
Gait:	
Posture:	

Central nervous system	
Orientation to • Time: • Place: • Person:	
Speech, e.g., stammering, etc.	

Any other observations during physical examination:

_____

_____

_____

_____

Signature of Student Nurse   **Signature of Supervisor**

Physical Assessment – 3
Demographic Data

Name:	
Age:	
Gender:	
Address:	
Religion:	
Education:	
Occupation:	
Marital status:	
Informant:	
Date of admission:	
MRD No.:	
Diagnosis:	

Physical Assessment

Vital signs	
Temperature:	
Pulse rate:	
Respiratory rate:	
Blood pressure:	
General appearances	
Height = ft. inches, Weight = kg.	
Head	
Shape, scalp	
Hair	
Color, texture	
Eyes	
Eye brows:	
Eyelashes:	
Eyelids:	
Eyeballs:	
Conjunctiva:	
Pupil:	
Lens:	
Vision:	

Ears	
External ears:	
Hearing:	
Any other observations:	
Nose	
External nares:	
Nostrils:	
Any other observations:	
Mouth	
Lips:	
Tongue:	
Gums:	
Teeth:	
Neck	
Range of motion (ROM):	
Thyroid:	
Lymph nodes:	
Skin	
Color, tone	
Any other observations:	
Upper extremities	
Left arm/hand:	
Right arm/hand:	
Lower extremities	
Left leg/feet:	
Right leg/feet:	
Cardiovascular system	
Heart sounds (Inspection, Palpation, Percussion, Auscultation):	
Respiratory system	
Respiratory sounds (Inspection, Palpation, Percussion, Auscultation):	
Gastrointestinal system	
Appetite:	
Bowel habits:	
Abdominal finding (Inspection, Palpation, Percussion, Auscultation):	

Physical Assessment

Genitourinary system	
Musculoskeletal system	
Gait:	
Posture:	
Central nervous system	
Orientation to • Time: • Place: • Person:	
Speech, e.g., stammering, etc.	

Any other observations during physical examination:

_____

_____

_____

_____

Signature of Student Nurse   **Signature of Supervisor**

Physical Assessment – 4
Demographic Data

Name:	
Age:	
Gender:	
Address:	
Religion:	
Education:	
Occupation:	
Marital status:	
Informant:	
Date of admission:	
MRD No.:	
Diagnosis:	

Physical Assessment

Vital signs	
Temperature:	
Pulse rate:	
Respiratory rate:	
Blood pressure:	
General appearances	
Height = ft. inches, Weight = kg.	
Head	
Shape, scalp	
Hair	
Color, texture	
Eyes	
Eye brows:	
Eyelashes:	
Eyelids:	
Eyeballs:	
Conjunctiva:	
Pupil:	
Lens:	
Vision:	

Ears	
External ears:	
Hearing:	
Any other observations:	
Nose	
External nares:	
Nostrils:	
Any other observations:	
Mouth	
Lips:	
Tongue:	
Gums:	
Teeth:	
Neck	
Range of motion (ROM):	
Thyroid:	
Lymph nodes:	
Skin	
Color, tone	
Any other observations:	
Upper extremities	
Left arm/hand:	
Right arm/hand:	
Lower extremities	
Left leg/feet:	
Right leg/feet:	
Cardiovascular system	
Heart sounds (Inspection, Palpation, Percussion, Auscultation):	
Respiratory system	
Respiratory sounds (Inspection, Palpation, Percussion, Auscultation):	
Gastrointestinal system	
Appetite:	
Bowel habits:	
Abdominal finding (Inspection, Palpation, Percussion, Auscultation):	

Genitourinary system	
Musculoskeletal system	
Gait:	
Posture:	
Central nervous system	
Orientation to • Time: • Place: • Person:	
Speech, e.g., stammering, etc.	

Any other observations during physical examination:

___

___

___

___

Signature of Student Nurse **Signature of Supervisor**

Physical Assessment – 5
Demographic Data

Name:	
Age:	
Gender:	
Address:	
Religion:	
Education:	
Occupation:	
Marital status:	
Informant:	
Date of admission:	
MRD No.:	
Diagnosis:	

Physical Assessment

Vital signs	
Temperature:	
Pulse rate:	
Respiratory rate:	
Blood pressure:	
General appearances	
Height = ft. inches, Weight = kg.	
Head	
Shape, scalp	
Hair	
Color, texture	
Eyes	
Eye brows:	
Eyelashes:	
Eyelids:	
Eyeballs:	
Conjunctiva:	
Pupil:	
Lens:	
Vision:	

Ears	
External ears:	
Hearing:	
Any other observations:	
Nose	
External nares:	
Nostrils:	
Any other observations:	
Mouth	
Lips:	
Tongue:	
Gums:	
Teeth:	
Neck	
Range of motion (ROM):	
Thyroid:	
Lymph nodes:	
Skin	
Color, tone	
Any other observations:	
Upper extremities	
Left arm/hand:	
Right arm/hand:	
Lower extremities	
Left leg/feet:	
Right leg/feet:	
Cardiovascular system	
Heart sounds (Inspection, Palpation, Percussion, Auscultation):	
Respiratory system	
Respiratory sounds (Inspection, Palpation, Percussion, Auscultation):	
Gastrointestinal system	
Appetite:	
Bowel habits:	
Abdominal finding (Inspection, Palpation, Percussion, Auscultation):	

Physical Assessment

Genitourinary system	
Musculoskeletal system	
Gait:	
Posture:	
Central nervous system	
Orientation to • Time: • Place: • Person:	
Speech, e.g., stammering, etc.	

Any other observations during physical examination:

_____

_____

_____

_____

Signature of Student Nurse   **Signature of Supervisor**

MENTAL STATUS EXAMINATION (MSE)

Mental Status Examination (MSE): The mental status examination includes overall assessment made during the clinical examination, including the specific tests based on the needs of the patient. Multiple cognitive functions may be tested, including attention, executive functioning, memory, orientation, thought content, thought processes. This tool is meant to diagnostic for any mental status disorder. Each must be interpreted in the context of examiner's observation. The mental status examination is used in differentiating between a variety of systemic conditions, like neurologic and psychiatric disorders ranging from delirium and dementia to mood disorder, schizophrenia and other neurosis or psychotic conditions.

MSE – 1
Demographic Data

Name:	
Age:	
Gender:	
Address:	
Religion:	
Education:	
Occupation:	
Marital status:	
Informant:	
Date of admission:	
MRD No.:	
Diagnosis:	

Mental Status Examination (MSE)

I. General Appearance and Behavior (GAAB):

• Facial expression (e.g., anxiety, pleasure, confidence, blunted, pleasant):	
• Posture (stooped, stiff, guarded, normal):	
• Mannerisms (stereotype, negativism, tics, normal):	
• Eye to eye contact (maintained or not):	
• Rapport (built easily or not built or built with difficulty):	
• Consciousness (conscious or drowsy or unconscious):	
• Behavior (includes social behavior, e.g., overfriendly, disinterested, preoccupied, aggressive, normal):	
• Dressing and grooming – well-dressed/appropriate/ inappropriate (to season and situation)/neat and tidy/dirty:	
• Physical features: Looks of one's age/look older/younger than his or her age/underweight/overweight/physical deformity:	

II. Psychomotor Activity:

• Increased/decreased/compulsive/ echopraxia/stereotypy/negativism/ automatic obedience:	

III. Speech:

• One sample of speech (verbatim in 2 or 3 sentences):	
• Coherence—Coherent/incoherent:	
• Relevance (answer the questions appropriately)—Relevant/irrelevant:	
• Volume (soft, loud or normal):	
• Tone (high pitch, low pitch, or normal/ monotonous):	
• Manner—Excessive formal/relaxed/ inappropriately familiar:	
• Reaction time (time taken to answer the question)—Increased, decreased or normal:	

IV. Thought:

• Form of thought/formal thought disorder—not understandable/normal/circumstantiality/tangentiality/neologism/word salad/preservation/ambivalence:	
• Stream of thought/flow of thought—pressure of speech/flight of ideas/thought retardation/mutism/aphonia/thought block/Clang association:	
• Content of thought	
– Delusions (specify type and give example)—Persecutory/delusion of reference/delusions of influence or passivity/hypochondriacal delusions/delusions of grandeur/nihilistic—Derealization/depersonalization/delusions of infidelity	
– Obsession:	
– Phobia:	
– Preoccupation:	
– Fantasy—Creative/day dreaming:	

V. Mood (subjective) and Affect (objective):

Student nurse: **Client:**

• Appropriate/inappropriate (Relevance to situation and thought congruent):	
• Pleasurable affect—Euphoria/elation/exaltation/ecstasy:	
• Other affects—Anxiety/fear/panic/free floating anxiety/apathy/aggression/moods swing/emotional liability:	

VI. Disorders Perception:

• Illusion:	
• Hallucinations (specify type and give example)—auditory/visual/olfactory/gustatory/tactile:	

VII. Cognitive Functions:

• Attention and concentration:	
Method of testing (asking to list the days of week forward and backward):	
Serial subtractions (100-7):	
• **Memory:**	
Immediate (Teach an address and after 5 mts. Asking for recall):	
Recent memory (24 hrs. recall):	
Remote (Asking for dates of birth or events which are occurred long back):	
• **Orientation**	
Time—Approximately without looking at the watch, what time is it?	
Place—Where he/she is now?	
Person—Who has accompanied him or her?	

Mental Status Examination (MSE)

• **Abstraction:**	
Give a proverb and ask the inner meaning (e.g., feathers of a bird flock together/rolling stones gather no mass):	
Intelligence and general information: Test by carry over sums/similarities and differences/ and general information/digit score test	
• **Judgment:**	
Personal (future plans):	
Social (perception of the society):	
Test (present a situation and ask their response to the situation):	
• **Insight:**	
Complete denial of illness:	
Slight awareness of being sick:	
Awareness of being sick attribute it to external/physical factor:	
Awareness of being sick, but due to something unknown in himself:	
Intellectual insight:	
True emotional insight:	

Signature of Student Nurse   **Signature of Supervisor**

MSE – 2

Demographic Data

Name:	
Age:	
Gender:	
Address:	
Religion:	
Education:	
Occupation:	
Marital status:	
Informant:	
Date of admission:	
MRD No.:	
Diagnosis:	

Mental Status Examination (MSE)

I. General Appearance and Behavior (GAAB):

• Facial expression (e.g., anxiety, pleasure, confidence, blunted, pleasant):	
• Posture (stooped, stiff, guarded, normal):	
• Mannerisms (stereotype, negativism, tics, normal):	
• Eye to eye contact (maintained or not):	
• Rapport (built easily or not built or built with difficulty):	
• Consciousness (conscious or drowsy or unconscious):	
• Behavior (includes social behavior, e.g., overfriendly, disinterested, preoccupied, aggressive, normal):	
• Dressing and grooming – well-dressed/appropriate/inappropriate (to season and situation)/neat and tidy/dirty:	
• Physical features: Looks of one's age/look older/younger than his or her age/underweight/overweight/physical deformity:	

II. Psychomotor Activity:

• Increased/decreased/compulsive/ echopraxia/stereotypy/negativism/ automatic obedience:	

III. Speech:

• One sample of speech (verbatim in 2 or 3 sentences):	
• Coherence—Coherent/incoherent:	
• Relevance (answer the questions appropriately)—Relevant/irrelevant:	
• Volume (soft, loud or normal):	
• Tone (high pitch, low pitch, or normal/ monotonous):	
• Manner—Excessive formal/relaxed/ inappropriately familiar:	
• Reaction time (time taken to answer the question)—Increased, decreased or normal:	

IV. Thought:

• Form of thought/formal thought disorder—not understandable/normal/circumstantiality/tangentiality/neologism/word salad/preservation/ambivalence:	
• Stream of thought/flow of thought—pressure of speech/flight of ideas/thought retardation/mutism/aphonia/thought block/Clang association:	
• Content of thought	
– Delusions (specify type and give example)—Persecutory/delusion of reference/delusions of influence or passivity/hypochondriacal delusions/delusions of grandeur/nihilistic—Derealization/depersonalization/delusions of infidelity	
– Obsession:	
– Phobia:	
– Preoccupation:	
– Fantasy—Creative/day dreaming:	

V. Mood (subjective) and Affect (objective):

Student nurse:　　　　　　　　　　　　　　　　　　　**Client:**

• Appropriate/inappropriate (Relevance to situation and thought congruent):	
• Pleasurable affect—Euphoria/elation/exaltation/ecstasy:	
• Other affects—Anxiety/fear/panic/free floating anxiety/apathy/aggression/moods swing/emotional liability:	

VI. Disorders Perception:

• Illusion:	
• Hallucinations (specify type and give example)—auditory/visual/olfactory/gustatory/tactile:	

VII. Cognitive Functions:

• **Attention and concentration:**	
Method of testing (asking to list the days of week forward and backward):	
Serial subtractions (100-7):	
• **Memory:**	
Immediate (Teach an address and after 5 mts. Asking for recall):	
Recent memory (24 hrs. recall):	
Remote (Asking for dates of birth or events which are occurred long back):	
• **Orientation**	
Time—Approximately without looking at the watch, what time is it?	
Place—Where he/she is now?	
Person—Who has accompanied him or her?	

• **Abstraction:**	
Give a proverb and ask the inner meaning (e.g., feathers of a bird flock together/rolling stones gather no mass):	
Intelligence and general information: Test by carry over sums/similarities and differences/ and general information/digit score test	
• **Judgment:**	
Personal (future plans):	
Social (perception of the society):	
Test (present a situation and ask their response to the situation):	
• **Insight:**	
Complete denial of illness:	
Slight awareness of being sick:	
Awareness of being sick attribute it to external/physical factor:	
Awareness of being sick, but due to something unknown in himself:	
Intellectual insight:	
True emotional insight:	

Signature of Student Nurse   **Signature of Supervisor**

MSE – 3
Demographic Data

Name:	
Age:	
Gender:	
Address:	
Religion:	
Education:	
Occupation:	
Marital status:	
Informant:	
Date of admission:	
MRD No.:	
Diagnosis:	

Mental Status Examination (MSE)

I. General Appearance and Behavior (GAAB):

• Facial expression (e.g., anxiety, pleasure, confidence, blunted, pleasant):	
• Posture (stooped, stiff, guarded, normal):	
• Mannerisms (stereotype, negativism, tics, normal):	
• Eye to eye contact (maintained or not):	
• Rapport (built easily or not built or built with difficulty):	
• Consciousness (conscious or drowsy or unconscious):	
• Behavior (includes social behavior, e.g., overfriendly, disinterested, preoccupied, aggressive, normal):	
• Dressing and grooming – well-dressed/appropriate/ inappropriate (to season and situation)/neat and tidy/dirty:	
• Physical features: Looks of one's age/look older/younger than his or her age/underweight/overweight/physical deformity:	

II. Psychomotor Activity:

• Increased/decreased/compulsive/ echopraxia/stereotypy/negativism/ automatic obedience:	

III. Speech:

• One sample of speech (verbatim in 2 or 3 sentences):	
• Coherence—Coherent/incoherent:	
• Relevance (answer the questions appropriately)—Relevant/irrelevant:	
• Volume (soft, loud or normal):	
• Tone (high pitch, low pitch, or normal/ monotonous):	
• Manner—Excessive formal/relaxed/ inappropriately familiar:	
• Reaction time (time taken to answer the question)—Increased, decreased or normal:	

Mental Status Examination (MSE) | 51

IV. Thought:

• Form of thought/formal thought disorder—not understandable/normal/circumstantiality/tangentiality/neologism/word salad/preservation/ambivalence:	
• Stream of thought/flow of thought—pressure of speech/flight of ideas/thought retardation/mutism/aphonia/thought block/Clang association:	
• Content of thought	
– Delusions (specify type and give example)—Persecutory/delusion of reference/delusions of influence or passivity/hypochondriacal delusions/delusions of grandeur/nihilistic—Derealization/depersonalization/delusions of infidelity	
– Obsession:	
– Phobia:	
– Preoccupation:	
– Fantasy—Creative/day dreaming:	

V. Mood (subjective) and Affect (objective):

Student nurse: **Client:**

• Appropriate/inappropriate (Relevance to situation and thought congruent):	
• Pleasurable affect—Euphoria/elation/exaltation/ecstasy:	
• Other affects—Anxiety/fear/panic/free floating anxiety/apathy/aggression/moods swing/emotional liability:	

VI. Disorders Perception:

• Illusion:	
• Hallucinations (specify type and give example)—auditory/visual/olfactory/gustatory/tactile:	

VII. Cognitive Functions:

• **Attention and concentration:**	
Method of testing (asking to list the days of week forward and backward):	
Serial subtractions (100-7):	
• **Memory:**	
Immediate (Teach an address and after 5 mts. Asking for recall):	
Recent memory (24 hrs. recall):	
Remote (Asking for dates of birth or events which are occurred long back):	
• **Orientation**	
Time—Approximately without looking at the watch, what time is it?	
Place—Where he/she is now?	
Person—Who has accompanied him or her?	

Mental Status Examination (MSE)

• **Abstraction:**	
Give a proverb and ask the inner meaning (e.g., feathers of a bird flock together/rolling stones gather no mass):	
Intelligence and general information: Test by carry over sums/similarities and differences/ and general information/digit score test	
• **Judgment:**	
Personal (future plans):	
Social (perception of the society):	
Test (present a situation and ask their response to the situation):	
• **Insight:**	
Complete denial of illness:	
Slight awareness of being sick:	
Awareness of being sick attribute it to external/physical factor:	
Awareness of being sick, but due to something unknown in himself:	
Intellectual insight:	
True emotional insight:	

Signature of Student Nurse   **Signature of Supervisor**

MSE – 4

Demographic Data

Name:	
Age:	
Gender:	
Address:	
Religion:	
Education:	
Occupation:	
Marital status:	
Informant:	
Date of admission:	
MRD No.:	
Diagnosis:	

Mental Status Examination (MSE)

I. General Appearance and Behavior (GAAB):

• Facial expression (e.g., anxiety, pleasure, confidence, blunted, pleasant):	
• Posture (stooped, stiff, guarded, normal):	
• Mannerisms (stereotype, negativism, tics, normal):	
• Eye to eye contact (maintained or not):	
• Rapport (built easily or not built or built with difficulty):	
• Consciousness (conscious or drowsy or unconscious):	
• Behavior (includes social behavior, e.g., overfriendly, disinterested, preoccupied, aggressive, normal):	
• Dressing and grooming – well-dressed/appropriate/inappropriate (to season and situation)/neat and tidy/dirty:	
• Physical features: Looks of one's age/look older/younger than his or her age/underweight/overweight/physical deformity:	

II. Psychomotor Activity:

• Increased/decreased/compulsive/ echopraxia/stereotypy/negativism/ automatic obedience:	

III. Speech:

• One sample of speech (verbatim in 2 or 3 sentences):	
• Coherence—Coherent/incoherent:	
• Relevance (answer the questions appropriately)—Relevant/irrelevant:	
• Volume (soft, loud or normal):	
• Tone (high pitch, low pitch, or normal/ monotonous):	
• Manner—Excessive formal/relaxed/ inappropriately familiar:	
• Reaction time (time taken to answer the question)—Increased, decreased or normal:	

IV. Thought:

• Form of thought/formal thought disorder—not understandable/normal/circumstantiality/tangentiality/neologism/word salad/preservation/ambivalence:	
• Stream of thought/flow of thought—pressure of speech/flight of ideas/thought retardation/mutism/aphonia/thought block/Clang association:	
• Content of thought	
– Delusions (specify type and give example)—Persecutory/delusion of reference/delusions of influence or passivity/hypochondriacal delusions/delusions of grandeur/nihilistic—Derealization/depersonalization/delusions of infidelity	
– Obsession:	
– Phobia:	
– Preoccupation:	
– Fantasy—Creative/day dreaming:	

V. Mood (subjective) and Affect (objective):

Student nurse: **Client:**

• Appropriate/inappropriate (Relevance to situation and thought congruent):	
• Pleasurable affect—Euphoria/elation/exaltation/ecstasy:	
• Other affects—Anxiety/fear/panic/free floating anxiety/apathy/aggression/moods swing/emotional liability:	

VI. Disorders Perception:

• Illusion:	
• Hallucinations (specify type and give example)—auditory/visual/olfactory/gustatory/tactile:	

VII. Cognitive Functions:

• **Attention and concentration:**	
Method of testing (asking to list the days of week forward and backward):	
Serial subtractions (100-7):	
• **Memory:**	
Immediate (Teach an address and after 5 mts. Asking for recall):	
Recent memory (24 hrs. recall):	
Remote (Asking for dates of birth or events which are occurred long back):	
• **Orientation**	
Time—Approximately without looking at the watch, what time is it?	
Place—Where he/she is now?	
Person—Who has accompanied him or her?	

• **Abstraction:**	
Give a proverb and ask the inner meaning (e.g., feathers of a bird flock together/rolling stones gather no mass):	
Intelligence and general information: Test by carry over sums/similarities and differences/ and general information/digit score test	
• **Judgment:**	
Personal (future plans):	
Social (perception of the society):	
Test (present a situation and ask their response to the situation):	
• **Insight:**	
Complete denial of illness:	
Slight awareness of being sick:	
Awareness of being sick attribute it to external/physical factor:	
Awareness of being sick, but due to something unknown in himself:	
Intellectual insight:	
True emotional insight:	

Signature of Student Nurse   **Signature of Supervisor**

MSE – 5
Demographic Data

Name:	
Age:	
Gender:	
Address:	
Religion:	
Education:	
Occupation:	
Marital status:	
Informant:	
Date of admission:	
MRD No.:	
Diagnosis:	

Mental Status Examination (MSE)

I. General Appearance and Behavior (GAAB):

• Facial expression (e.g., anxiety, pleasure, confidence, blunted, pleasant):	
• Posture (stooped, stiff, guarded, normal):	
• Mannerisms (stereotype, negativism, tics, normal):	
• Eye to eye contact (maintained or not):	
• Rapport (built easily or not built or built with difficulty):	
• Consciousness (conscious or drowsy or unconscious):	
• Behavior (includes social behavior, e.g., overfriendly, disinterested, preoccupied, aggressive, normal):	
• Dressing and grooming – well-dressed/appropriate/ inappropriate (to season and situation)/neat and tidy/dirty:	
• Physical features: Looks of one's age/look older/younger than his or her age/underweight/overweight/physical deformity:	

II. Psychomotor Activity:

• Increased/decreased/compulsive/echopraxia/stereotypy/negativism/automatic obedience:	

III. Speech:

• One sample of speech (verbatim in 2 or 3 sentences):	
• Coherence—Coherent/incoherent:	
• Relevance (answer the questions appropriately)—Relevant/irrelevant:	
• Volume (soft, loud or normal):	
• Tone (high pitch, low pitch, or normal/monotonous):	
• Manner—Excessive formal/relaxed/inappropriately familiar:	
• Reaction time (time taken to answer the question)—Increased, decreased or normal:	

IV. Thought:

• Form of thought/formal thought disorder—not understandable/normal/circumstantiality/tangentiality/neologism/word salad/preservation/ambivalence:	
• Stream of thought/flow of thought—pressure of speech/flight of ideas/thought retardation/mutism/aphonia/thought block/Clang association:	
• Content of thought	
- Delusions (specify type and give example)—Persecutory/delusion of reference/delusions of influence or passivity/hypochondriacal delusions/delusions of grandeur/nihilistic—Derealization/depersonalization/delusions of infidelity	
- Obsession:	
- Phobia:	
- Preoccupation:	
- Fantasy—Creative/day dreaming:	

V. Mood (subjective) and Affect (objective):

Student nurse: **Client:**

• Appropriate/inappropriate (Relevance to situation and thought congruent):	
• Pleasurable affect—Euphoria/elation/exaltation/ecstasy:	
• Other affects—Anxiety/fear/panic/free floating anxiety/apathy/aggression/moods swing/emotional liability:	

VI. Disorders Perception:

• Illusion:	
• Hallucinations (specify type and give example)—auditory/visual/olfactory/gustatory/tactile:	

VII. Cognitive Functions:

• **Attention and concentration:**	
Method of testing (asking to list the days of week forward and backward):	
Serial subtractions (100-7):	

• **Memory:**	
Immediate (Teach an address and after 5 mts. Asking for recall):	
Recent memory (24 hrs. recall):	
Remote (Asking for dates of birth or events which are occurred long back):	

• **Orientation**	
Time—Approximately without looking at the watch, what time is it?	
Place—Where he/she is now?	
Person—Who has accompanied him or her?	

• **Abstraction:**	
Give a proverb and ask the inner meaning (e.g., feathers of a bird flock together/rolling stones gather no mass):	
Intelligence and general information: Test by carry over sums/similarities and differences/ and general information/digit score test	
• **Judgment:**	
Personal (future plans):	
Social (perception of the society):	
Test (present a situation and ask their response to the situation):	
• **Insight:**	
Complete denial of illness:	
Slight awareness of being sick:	
Awareness of being sick attribute it to external/physical factor:	
Awareness of being sick, but due to something unknown in himself:	
Intellectual insight:	
True emotional insight:	

Signature of Student Nurse   **Signature of Supervisor**

MINI-MENTAL STATUS EXAMINATION (MMSE)

A Mini-Mental State Examination (MMSE) is a set of 11 questions that doctors and other healthcare professionals commonly use to check for cognitive impairment (problems with thinking, communication, understanding and memory).

These 11-question tests five areas of cognitive function: orientation, registration, attention and calculation, recall, and language. The maximum score is 30.

MMSE – 1

Patient Name: _____

MRD No.: _____

Date: _____

Time: _____

Mini-Mental Status Examination (MMSE)

	Student nurses	*Patient response*	*Points*	*Patient score*
1.	**Orientation**			
1.1	What is the year?		1	
1.2	What is season?		1	
1.3	What is the date today?		1	
1.4	Which day is today?		1	
1.5	Which month?		1	
1.6	Which is your state?		1	
1.7	Country		1	
1.8	Which city is this?		1	
1.9	Name of this hospital		1	
1.10	Which floor is this ward?		1	
2.	**Attention and calculation**			
2.1	Spell word Apple		1	
2.2	Subtract 7 from 100 (if response is correct continue for 5 calculations)		1	
2.3	Subtract 7 from 93		1	
2.4	Subtract 7 from 86		1	
2.5	Subtract 7 from 79		1	
3.	**Registration**			
3.1	I will name three objects listen carefully 1. Apple 2. Table 3. Pen Now repeat the objects		3	
4.	**Recall**			
4.1	Now tell me all the objects which I had told you		3	
5.	**Language**			
5.1	What is the name of this (point towards some object around, e.g., pen in your hand)?		1	
5.2	What is the name of this (point towards some other object around)?		1	
5.3	Now repeat these 2 objects I showed you		1	
5.4	Now follow the command what I do example "raise right hand then raise left hand and rub with one another"		3	
5.5	Now I will write something on paper you read it and do the same. Example "close your eyes"		1	
5.6	Now write any sentence of your choice which contains subject and verb		1	
5.7	Now I will draw figure and you copy the exact design		1	
	Total		30	

Interpretation

- A score of 25 or higher is classed as normal.
- If the score is below 24, the result is usually considered to be abnormal, indicating possible cognitive impairment.

Signature of Supervisor

MMSE – 2

Patient Name: _____
MRD No.: _____
Date: _____
Time: _____

Mini-Mental Status Examination (MMSE)

	Student nurses	Patient response	Points	Patient score
1.	**Orientation**			
1.1	What is the year?		1	
1.2	What is season?		1	
1.3	What is the date today?		1	
1.4	Which day is today?		1	
1.5	Which month?		1	
1.6	Which is your state?		1	
1.7	Country		1	
1.8	Which city is this?		1	
1.9	Name of this hospital		1	
1.10	Which floor is this ward?		1	
2.	**Attention and calculation**			
2.1	Spell word Apple		1	
2.2	Subtract 7 from 100 (if response is correct continue for 5 calculations)		1	
2.3	Subtract 7 from 93		1	
2.4	Subtract 7 from 86		1	
2.5	Subtract 7 from 79		1	
3.	**Registration**			
3.1	I will name three objects listen carefully 1. Apple 2. Table 3. Pen Now repeat the objects		3	
4.	**Recall**			
4.1	Now tell me all the objects which I had told you		3	
5.	**Language**			
5.1	What is the name of this (point towards some object around, e.g., pen in your hand)?		1	
5.2	What is the name of this (point towards some other object around)?		1	
5.3	Now repeat these 2 objects I showed you		1	
5.4	Now follow the command what I do example "raise right hand then raise left hand and rub with one another"		3	
5.5	Now I will write something on paper you read it and do the same. Example "close your eyes"		1	
5.6	Now write any sentence of your choice which contains subject and verb		1	
5.7	Now I will draw figure and you copy the exact design		1	
	Total		30	

Interpretation

- A score of 25 or higher is classed as normal.
- If the score is below 24, the result is usually considered to be abnormal, indicating possible cognitive impairment.

Signature of Supervisor

MMSE – 3

Patient Name: _____

MRD No.: _____

Date: _____

Time: _____

Mini-Mental Status Examination (MMSE)

	Student nurses	Patient response	Points	Patient score
1.	**Orientation**			
1.1	What is the year?		1	
1.2	What is season?		1	
1.3	What is the date today?		1	
1.4	Which day is today?		1	
1.5	Which month?		1	
1.6	Which is your state?		1	
1.7	Country		1	
1.8	Which city is this?		1	
1.9	Name of this hospital		1	
1.10	Which floor is this ward?		1	
2.	**Attention and calculation**			
2.1	Spell word Apple		1	
2.2	Subtract 7 from 100 (if response is correct continue for 5 calculations)		1	
2.3	Subtract 7 from 93		1	
2.4	Subtract 7 from 86		1	
2.5	Subtract 7 from 79		1	
3.	**Registration**			
3.1	I will name three objects listen carefully 1. Apple 2. Table 3. Pen Now repeat the objects		3	
4.	**Recall**			
4.1	Now tell me all the objects which I had told you		3	
5.	**Language**			
5.1	What is the name of this (point towards some object around, e.g., pen in your hand)?		1	
5.2	What is the name of this (point towards some other object around)?		1	
5.3	Now repeat these 2 objects I showed you		1	
5.4	Now follow the command what I do example "raise right hand then raise left hand and rub with one another"		3	
5.5	Now I will write something on paper you read it and do the same. Example "close your eyes"		1	
5.6	Now write any sentence of your choice which contains subject and verb		1	
5.7	Now I will draw figure and you copy the exact design		1	
	Total		30	

Interpretation

- A score of 25 or higher is classed as normal.
- If the score is below 24, the result is usually considered to be abnormal, indicating possible cognitive impairment.

Signature of Supervisor

MMSE – 4

Patient Name: _____

MRD No.: _____

Date: _____

Time: _____

Mini-Mental Status Examination (MMSE)

	Student nurses	*Patient response*	*Points*	*Patient score*
1.	**Orientation**			
1.1	What is the year?		1	
1.2	What is season?		1	
1.3	What is the date today?		1	
1.4	Which day is today?		1	
1.5	Which month?		1	
1.6	Which is your state?		1	
1.7	Country		1	
1.8	Which city is this?		1	
1.9	Name of this hospital		1	
1.10	Which floor is this ward?		1	
2.	**Attention and calculation**			
2.1	Spell word Apple		1	
2.2	Subtract 7 from 100 (if response is correct continue for 5 calculations)		1	
2.3	Subtract 7 from 93		1	
2.4	Subtract 7 from 86		1	
2.5	Subtract 7 from 79		1	
3.	**Registration**			
3.1	I will name three objects listen carefully 1. Apple 2. Table 3. Pen Now repeat the objects		3	
4.	**Recall**			
4.1	Now tell me all the objects which I had told you		3	
5.	**Language**			
5.1	What is the name of this (point towards some object around, e.g., pen in your hand)?		1	
5.2	What is the name of this (point towards some other object around)?		1	
5.3	Now repeat these 2 objects I showed you		1	
5.4	Now follow the command what I do example "raise right hand then raise left hand and rub with one another"		3	
5.5	Now I will write something on paper you read it and do the same. Example "close your eyes"		1	
5.6	Now write any sentence of your choice which contains subject and verb		1	
5.7	Now I will draw figure and you copy the exact design		1	
	Total		30	

Interpretation

- A score of 25 or higher is classed as normal.
- If the score is below 24, the result is usually considered to be abnormal, indicating possible cognitive impairment.

Signature of Supervisor

MMSE – 5

Patient Name: _____

MRD No.: _____

Date: _____

Time: _____

Mini-Mental Status Examination (MMSE)

	Student nurses	Patient response	Points	Patient score
1.	**Orientation**			
1.1	What is the year?		1	
1.2	What is season?		1	
1.3	What is the date today?		1	
1.4	Which day is today?		1	
1.5	Which month?		1	
1.6	Which is your state?		1	
1.7	Country		1	
1.8	Which city is this?		1	
1.9	Name of this hospital		1	
1.10	Which floor is this ward?		1	
2.	**Attention and calculation**			
2.1	Spell word Apple		1	
2.2	Subtract 7 from 100 (if response is correct continue for 5 calculations)		1	
2.3	Subtract 7 from 93		1	
2.4	Subtract 7 from 86		1	
2.5	Subtract 7 from 79		1	
3.	**Registration**			
3.1	I will name 3 objects listen carefully 1. Apple 2. Table 3. Pen Now repeat the objects		3	
4.	**Recall**			
4.1	Now tell me all the objects which I had told you		3	
5.	**Language**			
5.1	What is the name of this (point towards some object around, e.g., pen in your hand)?		1	
5.2	What is the name of this (point towards some other object around)?		1	
5.3	Now repeat these 2 objects I showed you		1	
5.4	Now follow the command what I do example "raise right hand then raise left hand and rub with one another"		3	
5.5	Now I will write something on paper you read it and do the same. Example "close your eyes"		1	
5.6	Now write any sentence of your choice which contains subject and verb		1	
5.7	Now I will draw figure and you copy the exact design		1	
	Total		30	

Interpretation

- A score of 25 or higher is classed as normal.
- If the score is below 24, the result is usually considered to be abnormal, indicating possible cognitive impairment.

Signature of Supervisor

NEUROLOGICAL EXAMINATION

Neurological Examination: A neurological exam, also called a neuro exam, is an assessment of a patient's nervous system. In this examination, some instruments can be used such as lights and reflex hammers. It usually does not cause any pain to the patient but little uncomfortableness may be experienced. In this examination, all twelve cranial nerves are being assessed for their normal function or any deviation.

Neurological Examination – 1

Name:	
Age:	
Gender:	
Address:	
Religion:	
Education:	
Occupation:	
Marital status:	
Informant:	
Date of admission:	
MRD No.:	
Diagnosis:	

1. **Level of consciousness:** Alert/Lethargic/Stuporous/Semi-Comatose, Comatose:
2. **Score on Glasgow Coma Scale:**

Behavior	Response		Score in patient
Eye opening response	Spontaneous—open with blinking at baseline	4 points	
	To verbal stimuli, command, speech	3 points	
	To pain only (not applied to face)	2 points	
	No response	1 point	
Verbal response	Oriented	5 points	
	Confused conversation, but able to answer questions	4 points	
	Inappropriate words	3 points	
	Incomprehensible speech	2 points	
	No response	1 point	
Motor response	Obeys commands for movement	6 points	
	Purposeful movement to painful stimulus	5 points	
	Withdraws in response to pain	4 points	
	Flexion in response to pain (decorticate posturing)	3 points	
	Extension response in response to pain (decerebrate posturing)	2 points	
	No response	1 point	
Total score	**Fully consensus** **Comatose patient** **Totally unconscious**	15 8 or less 3	

Interpretation:
The GCS is scored between 3 and 15, 3 being the worst and 15 the best. It is composed of three parameters: best eye response (E), best verbal response (V), and best motor response (M). The components of the GCS should be recorded individually, for example, E2V3M5 results in a GCS score of 10.

3. Mental Status Examination:

1. General Appearance and Behavior: _____
   _____
   _____

2. Speech: _____
   _____
   _____

3. Mood and Affect: _____
   _____
   _____

4. Perception: _____
   _____
   _____

5. Cognition: _____
   _____
   _____

6. Insight: _____
   _____
   _____

7. Judgment: _____
   _____
   _____

4. Cranial Nerve Function:

Cranial nerve testing and functioning

S. No.	Cranial nerve	Function	Test
i.	• Olfactory nerve	• Sense of smell	• Ask patient to occlude one nostril and close your eyes. • Present a stimulus such as coffee and ask the patient to identify the smell.
ii.	• Optic nerve	• Vision	• Visual acuity. • Color vision. • Visual field. • Pupillary response to light to test for an afferent pupillary defect.
iii.	• Oculomotor	• Ocular motility • Lid elevation • Pupillary constriction	• Routinely tested during examination with extraocular motility. • Supraduction. • Infraduction. • Adduction.
iv.	• Trochlear	• Ocular motility	• Routinely tested during examination with extraocular motility. Infraduction upon adduction. • Intorsion.
v.	• Trigeminal	• Facial sensation and muscles of mastication	• Test the distribution of V_1, V_2, and V_3 separately with a light touch with a cotton wisp to the forehead, upper cheek and jaw, respectively with the patients eye closed. Ask the patient to compare the sensation from right to left looking for any asymmetry. • Assess the motor function of V by feeling either side of the jaw, just inferior and anterior to the ear for the muscle contraction, while asking the patient to clench their teeth. • If indicated, the corneal reflex with a cotton wisp.

Neurological Examination

vi.	**Abducens**	• Ocular motility	• Routinely tested during examination with extraocular motility. • Abduction
vii.	**Facial**	• Muscles of facial expression • Taste to anterior 2/3 tongue	• Ask the patient to smile, raise their eye brows, frown, puff out their cheeks and squeeze their eye lids tightly together while looking for any asymmetry or weakness.
viii.	**Vestibulocochlear**	• Auditory and vestibular system	• Hearing can be grossly checked by rubbing your fingers together near patients ear and asking that if they can identify which ear hears the sound if they notice any asymmetry in the voice of sound.
ix.	**Glossopharyngeal**	• Palate • Elevation, gag reflux, swallowing • Speaking	• Ask the patient to open their mouth and say "AAHH" and look for any asymmetry in the palate or deviation in the uvula.
x.	**Vagus**		
xi.	**Accessory**	• Sternocleidomastoid and trapezius muscle	• Ask the patient to turn their head side to side and shrug their shoulders looking for any asymmetry or weakness.
xii.	**Hypoglossal**	• Muscle of action of tongue	• Ask the patient to stick their tongue out and note if it deviates to one side.

Olfactory Nerve:

Example:

Student Nurse: Mr. ABC close your eyes. (close/block the one nostril of patient with fingers of hand), ok now smell (some mint or coffee in hand).

Patients Response: Can't smell.

a. **Olfactory Nerve**

   Student Nurse: _____

   _____

   Patients Response: _____

b. **Optic Nerve:**

   Student Nurse: _____

   Patients Response: _____

c. **Oculomotor:**

   Student Nurse: _____

   Patients Response: _____

d. **Trigeminal Nerve (IV):**

   Student Nurse: _____

   Patients Response: _____

e. **Facial Nerve (VII):**
   Student Nurse: _____
   _____
   Patients Response: _____
   _____

f. **Auditory Nerve (VIII):**
   Student Nurse: _____
   _____
   Patients Response: _____
   _____

g. **Glossopharyngeal (IX) and Vagus (X) Nerves:**
   Student Nurse: _____
   _____
   Patients Response: _____
   _____

h. **Spinal Accessory Nerve (XI):**
   Student Nurse: _____
   _____
   Patients Response: _____
   _____
   _____

i. **Hypoglossal (XII) Nerve:**
   Student Nurse: _____
   _____
   _____
   Patients Response: _____
   _____

5. **Assessment of Motor Function:**

Muscle Power Scale

Score	Description
0	No contraction
1	Flicker or trace of contraction
2	Active movement, with gravity eliminated
3	Active movement against gravity
4	Active movement against gravity and resistance
5	Normal power

Student Nurse: _____

Patients Response: _____

Score of Motor Power: _____

6. **Assessment of Sensory Function:**

   a. **Touch:**

   Student Nurse: _____

   Patients Response: _____

   b. **Pain:**

   Student Nurse: _____

   Patients Response: _____

   c. **Temperature:**

   Student Nurse: _____

   Patients Response: _____

   d. **Position:**

   Student Nurse: _____

   Patients Response: _____

7. **Assessment of Cerebellar Function:**

   Finger-to-finger test/Finger to nose test/Patting test/Romberg test/Tandem walking test.

   Student Nurse: _____

   Patients Response: _____

Neurological Examination – 2

Name:	
Age:	
Gender:	
Address:	
Religion:	
Education:	
Occupation:	
Marital status:	
Informant:	
Date of admission:	
MRD No.:	
Diagnosis:	

1. **Level of consciousness:** Alert/Lethargic/Stuporous/Semi-Comatose, Comatose:
2. **Score on Glasgow Coma Scale:**

Behavior	Response		Score in patient
Eye opening response	Spontaneous—open with blinking at baseline	4 points	
	To verbal stimuli, command, speech	3 points	
	To pain only (not applied to face)	2 points	
	No response	1 point	
Verbal response	Oriented	5 points	
	Confused conversation, but able to answer questions	4 points	
	Inappropriate words	3 points	
	Incomprehensible speech	2 points	
	No response	1 point	
Motor response	Obeys commands for movement	6 points	
	Purposeful movement to painful stimulus	5 points	
	Withdraws in response to pain	4 points	
	Flexion in response to pain (decorticate posturing)	3 points	
	Extension response in response to pain (decerebrate posturing)	2 points	
	No response	1 point	
Total score	**Fully consensus** **Comatose patient** **Totally unconscious**	15 8 or less 3	
Interpretation: The GCS is scored between 3 and 15, 3 being the worst and 15 the best. It is composed of three parameters: best eye response (E), best verbal response (V), and best motor response (M). The components of the GCS should be recorded individually, for example, E2V3M5 results in a GCS score of 10.			

Neurological Examination

3. **Mental Status Examination:**
   1. General Appearance and Behavior: _____
      _____
      _____
   2. Speech: _____
      _____
      _____
   3. Mood and Affect: _____
      _____
      _____
   4. Perception: _____
      _____
      _____
   5. Cognition: _____
      _____
      _____
   6. Insight: _____
      _____
      _____
   7. Judgment: _____
      _____
      _____

4. **Cranial Nerve Function:**

Cranial nerve testing and functioning

S. No.	Cranial nerve	Function	Test
i.	• Olfactory nerve	• Sense of smell	• Ask patient to occlude one nostril and close your eyes. • Present a stimulus such as coffee and ask the patient to identify the smell.
ii.	• Optic nerve	• Vision	• Visual acuity. • Color vision. • Visual field. • Pupillary response to light to test for an afferent pupillary defect.
iii.	• Oculomotor	• Ocular motility • Lid elevation • Pupillary constriction	• Routinely tested during examination with extraocular motility. • Supraduction. • Infraduction. • Adduction.
iv.	• Trochlear	• Ocular motility	• Routinely tested during examination with extraocular motility. Infraduction upon adduction. • Intorsion.
v.	• Trigeminal	• Facial sensation and muscles of mastication	• Test the distribution of V_1, V_2, and V_3 separately with a light touch with a cotton wisp to the forehead, upper cheek and jaw, respectively with the patients eye closed. Ask the patient to compare the sensation from right to left looking for any asymmetry. • Assess the motor function of V by feeling either side of the jaw, just inferior and anterior to the ear for the muscle contraction, while asking the patient to clench their teeth. • If indicated, the corneal reflex with a cotton wisp.

vi.	• **Abducens**	• Ocular motility	• Routinely tested during examination with extraocular motility. • Abduction
vii.	• **Facial**	• Muscles of facial expression • Taste to anterior 2/3 tongue	• Ask the patient to smile, raise their eye brows, frown, puff out their cheeks and squeeze their eye lids tightly together while looking for any asymmetry or weakness.
viii.	• **Vestibulocochlear**	• Auditory and vestibular system	• Hearing can be grossly checked by rubbing your fingers together near patients ear and asking that if they can identify which ear hears the sound if they notice any asymmetry in the voice of sound.
ix	• **Glossopharyngeal**	• Palate • Elevation, gag reflux, swallowing • Speaking	• Ask the patient to open their mouth and say "AAHH" and look for any asymmetry in the palate or deviation in the uvula.
x.	• **Vagus**		
xi.	• **Accessory**	• Sternocleidomastoid and trapezius muscle	• Ask the patient to turn their head side to side and shrug their shoulders looking for any asymmetry or weakness.
xii.	• **Hypoglossal**	• Muscle of action of tongue	• Ask the patient to stick their tongue out and note if it deviates to one side.

a. Olfactory Nerve

  Student Nurse: _____

  _____

  Patients Response: _____

  _____

b. Optic Nerve:

  Student Nurse: _____

  _____

  Patients Response: _____

c. Oculomotor:

  Student Nurse: _____

  Patients Response: _____

d. Trigeminal Nerve (IV):

  Student Nurse: _____

  Patients Response: _____

e. **Facial Nerve (VII):**
   Student Nurse: _____

   Patients Response: _____

f. **Auditory Nerve (VIII):**
   Student Nurse: _____

   Patients Response: _____

g. **Glossopharyngeal (IX) and Vagus (X) Nerves:**
   Student Nurse: _____

   Patients Response: _____

h. **Spinal Accessory Nerve (XI):**
   Student Nurse: _____

   Patients Response: _____

i. **Hypoglossal (XII) Nerve:**
   Student Nurse: _____

   Patients Response: _____

5. **Assessment of Motor Function:**
   Muscle Power Scale

Score	Description
0	No contraction
1	Flicker or trace of contraction
2	Active movement, with gravity eliminated
3	Active movement against gravity
4	Active movement against gravity and resistance
5	Normal power

Student Nurse: _____

_____

Patients Response: _____

Score of Motor Power: _____

6. **Assessment of Sensory Function:**

   a. **Touch:**

   Student Nurse: _____

   Patients Response: _____

   b. **Pain:**

   Student Nurse: _____

   Patients Response: _____

   c. **Temperature:**

   Student Nurse: _____

   Patients Response: _____

   d. **Position:**

   Student Nurse: _____

   Patients Response: _____

7. **Assessment of Cerebellar Function:**

   Finger-to-finger test/Finger to nose test/Patting test/Romberg test/Tandem walking test.

   Student Nurse: _____

   Patients Response: _____

Neurological Examination – 3

Name:	
Age:	
Gender:	
Address:	
Religion:	
Education:	
Occupation:	
Marital status:	
Informant:	
Date of admission:	
MRD No.:	
Diagnosis:	

1. **Level of consciousness:** Alert/Lethargic/Stuporous/Semi-Comatose, Comatose:
2. **Score on Glasgow Coma Scale:**

Behavior	Response		Score in patient
Eye opening response	Spontaneous—open with blinking at baseline	4 points	
	To verbal stimuli, command, speech	3 points	
	To pain only (not applied to face)	2 points	
	No response	1 point	
Verbal response	Oriented	5 points	
	Confused conversation, but able to answer questions	4 points	
	Inappropriate words	3 points	
	Incomprehensible speech	2 points	
	No response	1 point	
Motor response	Obeys commands for movement	6 points	
	Purposeful movement to painful stimulus	5 points	
	Withdraws in response to pain	4 points	
	Flexion in response to pain (decorticate posturing)	3 points	
	Extension response in response to pain (decerebrate posturing)	2 points	
	No response	1 point	
Total score	**Fully consensus** **Comatose patient** **Totally unconscious**	15 8 or less 3	

Interpretation:
The GCS is scored between 3 and 15, 3 being the worst and 15 the best. It is composed of three parameters: best eye response (E), best verbal response (V), and best motor response (M). The components of the GCS should be recorded individually, for example, E2V3M5 results in a GCS score of 10.

3. Mental Status Examination:

1. General Appearance and Behavior: _____
   _____
   _____

2. Speech: _____
   _____
   _____

3. Mood and Affect: _____
   _____
   _____

4. Perception: _____
   _____
   _____

5. Cognition: _____
   _____
   _____

6. Insight: _____
   _____
   _____

7. Judgment: _____
   _____

4. Cranial Nerve Function:

Cranial nerve testing and functioning

S. No.	Cranial nerve	Function	Test
i.	• Olfactory nerve	• Sense of smell	• Ask patient to occlude one nostril and close your eyes. • Present a stimulus such as coffee and ask the patient to identify the smell.
ii.	• Optic nerve	• Vision	• Visual acuity. • Color vision. • Visual field. • Pupillary response to light to test for an afferent pupillary defect.
iii.	• Oculomotor	• Ocular motility • Lid elevation • Pupillary constriction	• Routinely tested during examination with extraocular motility. • Supraduction. • Infraduction. • Adduction.
iv.	• Trochlear	• Ocular motility	• Routinely tested during examination with extraocular motility. Infraduction upon adduction. • Intorsion.
v.	• Trigeminal	• Facial sensation and muscles of mastication	• Test the distribution of V_1, V_2, and V_3 separately with a light touch with a cotton wisp to the forehead, upper cheek and jaw, respectively with the patients eye closed. Ask the patient to compare the sensation from right to left looking for any asymmetry. • Assess the motor function of V by feeling either side of the jaw, just inferior and anterior to the ear for the muscle contraction, while asking the patient to clench their teeth. • If indicated, the corneal reflex with a cotton wisp.

vi.	• Abducens	• Ocular motility	• Routinely tested during examination with extraocular motility. • Abduction
vii.	• Facial	• Muscles of facial expression • Taste to anterior 2/3 tongue	• Ask the patient to smile, raise their eye brows, frown, puff out their cheeks and squeeze their eye lids tightly together while looking for any asymmetry or weakness.
viii.	• Vestibulocochlear	• Auditory and vestibular system	• Hearing can be grossly checked by rubbing your fingers together near patients ear and asking that if they can identify which ear hears the sound if they notice any asymmetry in the voice of sound.
ix	• Glossopharyngeal	• Palate • Elevation, gag reflux, swallowing • Speaking	• Ask the patient to open their mouth and say "AAHH" and look for any asymmetry in the palate or deviation in the uvula.
x.	• Vagus		
xi.	• Accessory	• Sternocleidomastoid and trapezius muscle	• Ask the patient to turn their head side to side and shrug their shoulders looking for any asymmetry or weakness.
xii.	• Hypoglossal	• Muscle of action of tongue	• Ask the patient to stick their tongue out and note if it deviates to one side.

a. **Olfactory Nerve**

   Student Nurse: _____

   _____

   _____

   Patients Response: _____

   _____

   _____

b. **Optic Nerve:**

   Student Nurse: _____

   _____

   Patients Response: _____

   _____

c. **Oculomotor:**

   Student Nurse: _____

   _____

   Patients Response: _____

   _____

d. **Trigeminal Nerve (IV):**

   Student Nurse: _____

   _____

   Patients Response: _____

   _____

e. **Facial Nerve (VII):**
   Student Nurse: _____
   _____

   Patients Response: _____
   _____

f. **Auditory Nerve (VIII):**
   Student Nurse: _____
   _____

   Patients Response: _____
   _____

g. **Glossopharyngeal (IX) and Vagus (X) Nerves:**
   Student Nurse: _____
   _____

   Patients Response: _____
   _____

h. **Spinal Accessory Nerve (XI):**
   Student Nurse: _____
   _____

   Patients Response: _____
   _____
   _____

i. **Hypoglossal (XII) Nerve:**
   Student Nurse: _____
   _____

   Patients Response: _____
   _____
   _____

5. **Assessment of Motor Function:**
   Muscle Power Scale

Score	Description
0	No contraction
1	Flicker or trace of contraction
2	Active movement, with gravity eliminated
3	Active movement against gravity
4	Active movement against gravity and resistance
5	Normal power

Student Nurse: _____

_____

Patients Response: _____

_____

Score of Motor Power: _____

_____

6. **Assessment of Sensory Function:**

   a. **Touch:**

   Student Nurse: _____

   _____

   Patients Response: _____

   _____

   b. **Pain:**

   Student Nurse: _____

   _____

   Patients Response: _____

   _____

   c. **Temperature:**

   Student Nurse: _____

   _____

   Patients Response: _____

   _____

   _____

   d. **Position:**

   Student Nurse: _____

   _____

   Patients Response: _____

   _____

7. **Assessment of Cerebellar Function:**

   Finger-to-finger test/Finger to nose test/Patting test/Romberg test/Tandem walking test.

   Student Nurse: _____

   _____

   Patients Response: _____

   _____

   _____

Neurological Examination – 4

Name:	
Age:	
Gender:	
Address:	
Religion:	
Education:	
Occupation:	
Marital status:	
Informant:	
Date of admission:	
MRD No.:	
Diagnosis:	

1. **Level of consciousness:** Alert/Lethargic/Stuporous/Semi-Comatose, Comatose:
2. **Score on Glasgow Coma Scale:**

Behavior	Response		Score in patient
Eye opening response	Spontaneous—open with blinking at baseline	4 points	
	To verbal stimuli, command, speech	3 points	
	To pain only (not applied to face)	2 points	
	No response	1 point	
Verbal response	Oriented	5 points	
	Confused conversation, but able to answer questions	4 points	
	Inappropriate words	3 points	
	Incomprehensible speech	2 points	
	No response	1 point	
Motor response	Obeys commands for movement	6 points	
	Purposeful movement to painful stimulus	5 points	
	Withdraws in response to pain	4 points	
	Flexion in response to pain (decorticate posturing)	3 points	
	Extension response in response to pain (decerebrate posturing)	2 points	
	No response	1 point	
Total score	**Fully consensus**	15	
	Comatose patient	8 or less	
	Totally unconscious	3	
Interpretation: The GCS is scored between 3 and 15, 3 being the worst and 15 the best. It is composed of three parameters: best eye response (E), best verbal response (V), and best motor response (M). The components of the GCS should be recorded individually, for example, E2V3M5 results in a GCS score of 10.			

3. Mental Status Examination:

1. General Appearance and Behavior: _____
   _____

2. Speech: _____
   _____

3. Mood and Affect: _____
   _____

4. Perception: _____
   _____

5. Cognition: _____
   _____

6. Insight: _____
   _____

7. Judgment: _____
   _____

4. Cranial Nerve Function:

Cranial nerve testing and functioning			
S. No.	Cranial nerve	Function	Test
i.	• Olfactory nerve	• Sense of smell	• Ask patient to occlude one nostril and close your eyes. • Present a stimulus such as coffee and ask the patient to identify the smell.
ii.	• Optic nerve	• Vision	• Visual acuity. • Color vision. • Visual field. • Pupillary response to light to test for an afferent pupillary defect.
iii.	• Oculomotor	• Ocular motility • Lid elevation • Pupillary constriction	• Routinely tested during examination with extraocular motility. • Supraduction. • Infraduction. • Adduction.
iv.	• Trochlear	• Ocular motility	• Routinely tested during examination with extraocular motility. Infraduction upon adduction. • Intorsion.
v.	• Trigeminal	• Facial sensation and muscles of mastication	• Test the distribution of V_1, V_2, and V_3 separately with a light touch with a cotton wisp to the forehead, upper cheek and jaw, respectively with the patients eye closed. Ask the patient to compare the sensation from right to left looking for any asymmetry. • Assess the motor function of V by feeling either side of the jaw, just inferior and anterior to the ear for the muscle contraction, while asking the patient to clench their teeth. • If indicated, the corneal reflex with a cotton wisp.

vi.	**Abducens**	Ocular motility	Routinely tested during examination with extraocular motility.
			Abduction
vii.	**Facial**	Muscles of facial expression	Ask the patient to smile, raise their eye brows, frown, puff out their cheeks and squeeze their eye lids tightly together while looking for any asymmetry or weakness.
		Taste to anterior 2/3 tongue	
viii.	**Vestibulocochlear**	Auditory and vestibular system	Hearing can be grossly checked by rubbing your fingers together near patients ear and asking that if they can identify which ear hears the sound if they notice any asymmetry in the voice of sound.
ix.	**Glossopharyngeal**	Palate	Ask the patient to open their mouth and say "AAHH" and look for any asymmetry in the palate or deviation in the uvula.
		Elevation, gag reflux, swallowing	
x.	**Vagus**	Speaking	
xi.	**Accessory**	Sternocleidomastoid and trapezius muscle	Ask the patient to turn their head side to side and shrug their shoulders looking for any asymmetry or weakness.
xii.	**Hypoglossal**	Muscle of action of tongue	Ask the patient to stick their tongue out and note if it deviates to one side.

a. **Olfactory Nerve**

   Student Nurse: _____
   _____

   Patients Response: _____
   _____

b. **Optic Nerve:**

   Student Nurse: _____
   _____

   Patients Response: _____
   _____

c. **Oculomotor:**

   Student Nurse: _____
   _____

   Patients Response: _____
   _____

d. **Trigeminal Nerve (IV):**

   Student Nurse: _____
   _____

   Patients Response: _____
   _____

e. **Facial Nerve (VII):**
   Student Nurse: _____

   Patients Response: _____

f. **Auditory Nerve (VIII):**
   Student Nurse: _____

   Patients Response: _____

g. **Glossopharyngeal (IX) and Vagus (X) Nerves:**
   Student Nurse: _____

   Patients Response: _____

h. **Spinal Accessory Nerve (XI):**
   Student Nurse: _____

   Patients Response: _____

i. **Hypoglossal (XII) Nerve:**
   Student Nurse: _____

   Patients Response: _____

5. **Assessment of Motor Function:**
   Muscle Power Scale

Score	Description
0	No contraction
1	Flicker or trace of contraction
2	Active movement, with gravity eliminated
3	Active movement against gravity
4	Active movement against gravity and resistance
5	Normal power

Student Nurse: _____

_____

_____

Patients Response: _____

_____

Score of Motor Power: _____

_____

6. **Assessment of Sensory Function:**
   a. **Touch:**
      Student Nurse: _____

      _____

      Patients Response: _____

      _____

   b. **Pain:**
      Student Nurse: _____

      _____

      Patients Response: _____

      _____

   c. **Temperature:**
      Student Nurse: _____

      _____

      Patients Response: _____

      _____

      _____

   d. **Position:**
      Student Nurse: _____

      _____

      Patients Response: _____

      _____

7. **Assessment of Cerebellar Function:**
   Finger-to-finger test/Finger to nose test/Patting test/Romberg test/Tandem walking test.

   Student Nurse: _____

   _____

   Patients Response: _____

   _____

   _____

Neurological Examination – 5

Name:	
Age:	
Gender:	
Address:	
Religion:	
Education:	
Occupation:	
Marital status:	
Informant:	
Date of admission:	
MRD No.:	
Diagnosis:	

1. **Level of consciousness:** Alert/Lethargic/Stuporous/Semi-Comatose, Comatose:
2. **Score on Glasgow Coma Scale:**

Behavior	Response		Score in patient
Eye opening response	Spontaneous—open with blinking at baseline	4 points	
	To verbal stimuli, command, speech	3 points	
	To pain only (not applied to face)	2 points	
	No response	1 point	
Verbal response	Oriented	5 points	
	Confused conversation, but able to answer questions	4 points	
	Inappropriate words	3 points	
	Incomprehensible speech	2 points	
	No response	1 point	
Motor response	Obeys commands for movement	6 points	
	Purposeful movement to painful stimulus	5 points	
	Withdraws in response to pain	4 points	
	Flexion in response to pain (decorticate posturing)	3 points	
	Extension response in response to pain (decerebrate posturing)	2 points	
	No response	1 point	
Total score	**Fully consensus** **Comatose patient** **Totally unconscious**	15 8 or less 3	
Interpretation: The GCS is scored between 3 and 15, 3 being the worst and 15 the best. It is composed of three parameters: best eye response (E), best verbal response (V), and best motor response (M). The components of the GCS should be recorded individually, for example, E2V3M5 results in a GCS score of 10.			

3. Mental Status Examination:

1. General Appearance and Behavior: _____
   _____
   _____

2. Speech: _____
   _____
   _____

3. Mood and Affect: _____
   _____
   _____

4. Perception: _____
   _____
   _____

5. Cognition: _____
   _____
   _____

6. Insight: _____
   _____
   _____

7. Judgment: _____
   _____
   _____

4. Cranial Nerve Function:

Cranial nerve testing and functioning

S. No.	Cranial nerve	Function	Test
i.	• Olfactory nerve	• Sense of smell	• Ask patient to occlude one nostril and close your eyes. • Present a stimulus such as coffee and ask the patient to identify the smell.
ii.	• Optic nerve	• Vision	• Visual acuity. • Color vision. • Visual field. • Pupillary response to light to test for an afferent pupillary defect.
iii.	• Oculomotor	• Ocular motility • Lid elevation • Pupillary constriction	• Routinely tested during examination with extraocular motility. • Supraduction. • Infraduction. • Adduction.
iv.	• Trochlear	• Ocular motility	• Routinely tested during examination with extraocular motility. Infraduction upon adduction. • Intorsion.
v.	• Trigeminal	• Facial sensation and muscles of mastication	• Test the distribution of V_1, V_2, and V_3 separately with a light touch with a cotton wisp to the forehead, upper cheek and jaw, respectively with the patients eye closed. Ask the patient to compare the sensation from right to left looking for any asymmetry. • Assess the motor function of V by feeling either side of the jaw, just inferior and anterior to the ear for the muscle contraction, while asking the patient to clench their teeth. • If indicated, the corneal reflex with a cotton wisp.

vi.	**Abducens**	• Ocular motility	• Routinely tested during examination with extraocular motility. • Abduction
vii.	**Facial**	• Muscles of facial expression • Taste to anterior 2/3 tongue	• Ask the patient to smile, raise their eye brows, frown, puff out their cheeks and squeeze their eye lids tightly together while looking for any asymmetry or weakness.
viii.	**Vestibulocochlear**	• Auditory and vestibular system	• Hearing can be grossly checked by rubbing your fingers together near patients ear and asking that if they can identify which ear hears the sound if they notice any asymmetry in the voice of sound.
ix.	**Glossopharyngeal**	• Palate • Elevation, gag reflux, swallowing • Speaking	• Ask the patient to open their mouth and say "AAHH" and look for any asymmetry in the palate or deviation in the uvula.
x.	**Vagus**		
xi.	**Accessory**	• Sternocleidomastoid and trapezius muscle	• Ask the patient to turn their head side to side and shrug their shoulders looking for any asymmetry or weakness.
xii.	**Hypoglossal**	• Muscle of action of tongue	• Ask the patient to stick their tongue out and note if it deviates to one side.

a. **Olfactory Nerve**

   Student Nurse: _____

   _____

   Patients Response: _____

   _____

b. **Optic Nerve:**

   Student Nurse: _____

   _____

   Patients Response: _____

   _____

c. **Oculomotor:**

   Student Nurse: _____

   Patients Response: _____

d. **Trigeminal Nerve (IV):**

   Student Nurse: _____

   Patients Response: _____

   _____

e. **Facial Nerve (VII):**
   Student Nurse: _____
   _____

   Patients Response: _____
   _____

f. **Auditory Nerve (VIII):**
   Student Nurse: _____
   _____

   Patients Response: _____
   _____

g. **Glossopharyngeal (IX) and Vagus (X) Nerves:**
   Student Nurse: _____
   _____

   Patients Response: _____
   _____

h. **Spinal Accessory Nerve (XI):**
   Student Nurse: _____
   _____

   Patients Response: _____
   _____

i. **Hypoglossal (XII) Nerve:**
   Student Nurse: _____
   _____

   Patients Response: _____
   _____

5. **Assessment of Motor Function:**

   Muscle Power Scale

Score	Description
0	No contraction
1	Flicker or trace of contraction
2	Active movement, with gravity eliminated
3	Active movement against gravity
4	Active movement against gravity and resistance
5	Normal power

Student Nurse: _____

_____

Patients Response: _____

Score of Motor Power: _____

6. **Assessment of Sensory Function:**

   a. **Touch:**

      Student Nurse: _____

      Patients Response: _____

   b. **Pain:**

      Student Nurse: _____

      Patients Response: _____

   c. **Temperature:**

      Student Nurse: _____

      Patients Response: _____

      _____

   d. **Position:**

      Student Nurse: _____

      Patients Response: _____

7. **Assessment of Cerebellar Function:**

   Finger-to-finger test/Finger to nose test/Patting test/Romberg test/Tandem walking test.

   Student Nurse: _____

   Patients Response: _____

   _____

PROCESS RECORDING

Process Recording: Process recording is the tool used for interaction with the patients with psychiatric illness. It helps the student nurse to develop communication and interviewing skill. There are various therapeutic ways of communication used in the process. The below is example of process recording carried out by psychiatric nurse student. *(Process Recording, a way of Therapeutic Communication between a Nurse and Patient with Psychiatric Illness. Bushra Mushtaq)*

Process Recording – 1

Demographic Data

Name:	
Age:	
Sex:	
Address:	
Religion:	
Education:	
Occupation:	
Marital status:	
Information source:	
Date of admission:	
MRD No.:	
Diagnosis:	

Presenting Complaints

According to patient:
-
-
-
-

According to attendant:
-
-
-

History of presenting complaints:

Aims and Objectives of Interview:
For patient:
-
-
-

For student nurse:
-
-
-

Interview

Day: 1st   Date: Time: Duration: Minutes

Student nurse and patient	Content of interaction (Verbal/non-verbal response of student nurse and patient)	Inference
Student Nurse: Patient:		
Student Nurse: Patient:		
Student Nurse: Patient:		
Student Nurse: Patient:		
Student Nurse: Patient:		
Student Nurse: Patient:		
Student Nurse: Patient:		
Student Nurse: Patient:		

Summarization:

Signature of Supervisor

Interview

Day: 2nd **Date:** **Time:** **Duration:** **Minutes**

Student nurse and patient	Content of interaction (Verbal/non-verbal response of student nurse and patient)	Inference
Student Nurse: Patient:		
Student Nurse: Patient:		
Student Nurse: Patient:		
Student Nurse: Patient:		
Student Nurse: Patient:		
Student Nurse: Patient:		
Student Nurse: Patient:		
Student Nurse: Patient:		

Summarization:

Signature of Supervisor

Process Recording – 2

Demographic Data

Name:	
Age:	
Sex:	
Address:	
Religion:	
Education:	
Occupation:	
Marital status:	
Information source:	
Date of admission:	
MRD No.:	
Diagnosis:	

Presenting Complaints

According to patient:
-
-
-
-

According to attendant:
-
-
-

History of presenting complaints:

Aims and Objectives of Interview:
For patient:
-
-
-

For student nurse:
-
-
-

Interview

Day: 1st **Date:** **Time:** **Duration:** **Minutes**

Student nurse and patient	Content of interaction (Verbal/non-verbal response of student nurse and patient)	Inference
Student Nurse: Patient:		
Student Nurse: Patient:		
Student Nurse: Patient:		
Student Nurse: Patient:		
Student Nurse: Patient:		
Student Nurse: Patient:		
Student Nurse: Patient:		
Student Nurse: Patient:		

Summarization:

Signature of Supervisor

Interview

Day: 2nd Date: Time: Duration: Minutes

Student nurse and patient	Content of interaction (Verbal/non-verbal response of student nurse and patient)	Inference
Student Nurse: Patient:		
Student Nurse: Patient:		
Student Nurse: Patient:		
Student Nurse: Patient:		
Student Nurse: Patient:		
Student Nurse: Patient:		
Student Nurse: Patient:		
Student Nurse: Patient:		

Summarization:

Signature of Supervisor

Process Recording – 3

Demographic Data

Name:	
Age:	
Sex:	
Address:	
Religion:	
Education:	
Occupation:	
Marital status:	
Information source:	
Date of admission:	
MRD No.:	
Diagnosis:	

Presenting Complaints

According to patient:
-
-
-
-

According to attendant:
-
-
-

History of presenting complaints:

Aims and Objectives of Interview:
For patient:
-
-
-

For student nurse:
-
-
-

Interview

Day: 1st **Date:** **Time:** **Duration:** **Minutes**

Student nurse and patient	Content of interaction (Verbal/non-verbal response of student nurse and patient)	Inference
Student Nurse: Patient:		
Student Nurse: Patient:		
Student Nurse: Patient:		
Student Nurse: Patient:		
Student Nurse: Patient:		
Student Nurse: Patient:		
Student Nurse: Patient:		
Student Nurse: Patient:		

Summarization:

Signature of Supervisor

Interview

Day: 2nd **Date:** **Time:** **Duration:** **Minutes**

Student nurse and patient	Content of interaction (Verbal/non-verbal response of student nurse and patient)	Inference
Student Nurse: Patient:		
Student Nurse: Patient:		
Student Nurse: Patient:		
Student Nurse: Patient:		
Student Nurse: Patient:		
Student Nurse: Patient:		
Student Nurse: Patient:		
Student Nurse: Patient:		

Summarization:

Signature of Supervisor

Process Recording – 4

Demographic Data

Name:	
Age:	
Sex:	
Address:	
Religion:	
Education:	
Occupation:	
Marital status:	
Information source:	
Date of admission:	
MRD No.:	
Diagnosis:	

Presenting Complaints

According to patient:
-
-
-
-

According to attendant:
-
-
-

History of presenting complaints:

Aims and Objectives of Interview:
For patient:
-
-
-

For student nurse:
-
-
-

Process Recording

Interview

Day: 1st   Date: Time: Duration: Minutes

Student nurse and patient	Content of interaction (Verbal/non-verbal response of student nurse and patient)	Inference
Student Nurse: Patient:		
Student Nurse: Patient:		
Student Nurse: Patient:		
Student Nurse: Patient:		
Student Nurse: Patient:		
Student Nurse: Patient:		
Student Nurse: Patient:		
Student Nurse: Patient:		

Summarization:

Signature of Supervisor

Interview

Day: 2nd   Date: Time: Duration: Minutes

Student nurse and patient	Content of interaction (Verbal/non-verbal response of student nurse and patient)	Inference
Student Nurse: Patient:		
Student Nurse: Patient:		
Student Nurse: Patient:		
Student Nurse: Patient:		
Student Nurse: Patient:		
Student Nurse: Patient:		
Student Nurse: Patient:		
Student Nurse: Patient:		

Summarization:

Signature of Supervisor

Process Recording – 5
Demographic Data

Name:	
Age:	
Sex:	
Address:	
Religion:	
Education:	
Occupation:	
Marital status:	
Information source:	
Date of admission:	
MRD No.:	
Diagnosis:	

Presenting Complaints

According to patient:
-
-
-
-

According to attendant:
-
-
-

History of presenting complaints:

Aims and Objectives of Interview:
For patient:
-
-
-

For student nurse:
-
-
-

Interview

Day: 1st **Date:** **Time:** **Duration:** **Minutes**

Student nurse and patient	Content of interaction (Verbal/non-verbal response of student nurse and patient)	Inference
Student Nurse: Patient:		
Student Nurse: Patient:		
Student Nurse: Patient:		
Student Nurse: Patient:		
Student Nurse: Patient:		
Student Nurse: Patient:		
Student Nurse: Patient:		
Student Nurse: Patient:		

Summarization:

Signature of Supervisor

Interview

Day: 2nd **Date:** **Time:** **Duration:** **Minutes**

Student nurse and patient	Content of interaction (Verbal/non-verbal response of student nurse and patient)	Inference
Student Nurse: Patient:		
Student Nurse: Patient:		
Student Nurse: Patient:		
Student Nurse: Patient:		
Student Nurse: Patient:		
Student Nurse: Patient:		
Student Nurse: Patient:		
Student Nurse: Patient:		

Summarization:

Signature of Supervisor

ECT (ELECTROCONVULSIVE THERAPY)

ECT (Electroconvulsive Therapy): Initially, it was Meduna who used pharmacological methods like intramuscular injection of camphor and pentylenetetrazole to induce seizure.

Electroconvulsive therapy was first given by Italian neuropsychiatrists Ugo Cerletti and Lucio Bini in 1938. They started inducing seizures with electricity and called it EST or electroshock therapy. Later this method of treatment came to be known as ECT or electroconvulsive therapy.

ECT (Electroconvulsive Therapy) – 1

Name:	
Age:	
Gender:	
Address:	
Religion:	
Education:	
Occupation:	
Marital status:	
Information source:	
Date of admission:	
MRD No.:	
Diagnosis:	

Present indication for ECT:

History of past ECT session:

Session:

Pre-Procedure Assessment

Blood Pressure _____ Heart Rate _____

Respiratory Rate _____ Body Temperature (F) _____

Any medication taken: _____ consent given by _____

During Procedure

Anesthesia used: _____

Dose: _____ route _____

Other medications used:

S. No.	Name of drug	Use	Dose	Route	Remarks

- ECT frequency given: _____
- Duration of seizers produced: _____
- Next session date (if given): _____

Post Procedure Care

- **Level of consciousness:** _____
- **Oriented to:**
  - **Time:** _____
  - **Place:** _____
  - **Person:** _____
- Any side effects produced:
  - _____
  - _____
  - _____
  - _____

Education given to patient and attendant:

Remarks:

Signature of Student **Signature of Incharge ECT**

ECT (Electroconvulsive Therapy) – 2

Name:	
Age:	
Gender:	
Address:	
Religion:	
Education:	
Occupation:	
Marital status:	
Information source:	
Date of admission:	
MRD No.:	
Diagnosis:	

Present indication for ECT:

History of past ECT session:

Session:

Pre-Procedure Assessment

Blood Pressure _____ Heart Rate _____

Respiratory Rate _____ Body Temperature (F) _____

Any medication taken: _____ consent given by _____

During Procedure

Anesthesia used: _____

Dose: _____ route _____

Other medications used:

S. No	Name of drug	Use	Dose	Route	Remarks

- ECT frequency given: _____
- Duration of seizers produced: _____
- Next session date (if given): _____

Post Procedure Care

- **Level of consciousness:** _____
- **Oriented to:**
  - **Time:** _____
  - **Place:** _____
  - **Person:** _____
- **Any side effects produced:**
  - _____
  - _____
  - _____
  - _____

Education given to patient and attendant:

Remarks:

Signature of Student   **Signature of Incharge ECT**

ECT (Electroconvulsive Therapy) – 3

Name:	
Age:	
Gender:	
Address:	
Religion:	
Education:	
Occupation:	
Marital status:	
Information source:	
Date of admission:	
MRD No.:	
Diagnosis:	

Present indication for ECT:

History of past ECT session:

Session:

Pre-Procedure Assessment

Blood Pressure _____ Heart Rate _____

Respiratory Rate _____ Body Temperature (F) _____

Any medication taken: _____ consent given by _____

During Procedure

Anesthesia used: _____

Dose: _____ route _____

Other medications used:

S. No	Name of drug	Use	Dose	Route	Remarks

- ECT frequency given: _____
- Duration of seizers produced: _____
- Next session date (if given): _____

Post Procedure Care

- **Level of consciousness:** _____
- **Oriented to:**
    - **Time:** _____
    - **Place:** _____
    - **Person:** _____
- **Any side effects produced:**
    - _____
    - _____
    - _____
    - _____

Education given to patient and attendant:

Remarks:

Signature of Student   **Signature of Incharge ECT**

ECT (Electroconvulsive Therapy) – 4

Name:	
Age:	
Gender:	
Address:	
Religion:	
Education:	
Occupation:	
Marital status:	
Information source:	
Date of admission:	
MRD No.:	
Diagnosis:	

Present indication for ECT:

History of past ECT session:

Session:

Pre-Procedure Assessment

Blood Pressure _____ Heart Rate _____

Respiratory Rate _____ Body Temperature (F) _____

Any medication taken: _____ consent given by _____

During Procedure

Anesthesia used: _____

Dose: _____ route _____

Other medications used:

S. No	Name of drug	Use	Dose	Route	Remarks

- ECT frequency given: _____
- Duration of seizers produced: _____
- Next session date (if given): _____

Post Procedure Care
- **Level of consciousness:** _____
- **Oriented to:**
    - Time: _____
    - Place: _____
    - Person: _____
- **Any side effects produced:**
    - _____
    - _____
    - _____
    - _____

Education given to patient and attendant:

Remarks:

Signature of Student   **Signature of Incharge ECT**

ECT (Electroconvulsive Therapy) – 5

Name:	
Age:	
Gender:	
Address:	
Religion:	
Education:	
Occupation:	
Marital status:	
Information source:	
Date of admission:	
MRD No.:	
Diagnosis:	

Present indication for ECT:

History of past ECT session:

Session:

Pre-Procedure Assessment

Blood Pressure _____ Heart Rate _____

Respiratory Rate _____ Body Temperature (F) _____

Any medication taken: _____ consent given by _____

During Procedure

Anesthesia used: _____

Dose: _____ route _____

Other medications used:

S. No	Name of drug	Use	Dose	Route	Remarks

- ECT frequency given: _____
- Duration of seizers produced: _____
- Next session date (if given): _____

Post Procedure Care
- **Level of consciousness:** _____
- **Oriented to:**
  - Time: _____
  - Place: _____
  - Person: _____
- **Any side effects produced:**
  - _____
  - _____
  - _____
  - _____

Education given to patient and attendant:
Remarks:

Signature of Student **Signature of Incharge ECT**

THERAPIES

Therapy: Therapy is a treatment modality used to treat mental and emotional problems. There are various types of therapies used in psychiatric nursing for mentally ill patients. Therapies are given by professionally trained therapist. Various psychological therapies include: Therapeutic community (milieu therapy), psychotherapy-individual: psychoanalytical, cognitive and supportive, family, group, behavioral, Play, psychodrama, music, dance, recreational and light therapy, relaxation therapies: Yoga, meditation, biofeedback.

Therapy – 1

Name:	
Age:	
Sex:	
Address:	
Religion:	
Education:	
Occupation:	
Marital status:	
Informant:	
Date of admission:	
MRD No.:	
Diagnosis:	

Therapy Attended: _____ **Session:** _____

Date: _____ **Duration (in mints):** _____

Steps of Procedure: _____

_____

_____

_____

_____

_____

_____

_____

Summary: _____

_____

_____

_____

Signature of Student   **Signature of Therapist**

Therapy – 2

Name:	
Age:	
Sex:	
Address:	
Religion:	
Education:	
Occupation:	
Marital status:	
Informant:	
Date of admission:	
MRD No.:	
Diagnosis:	

Therapy Attended: _____ **Session:** _____

Date: _____ **Duration (in mints):** _____

Steps of Procedure: _____

_____

_____

_____

_____

_____

_____

_____

Summary: _____

_____

_____

Signature of Student   **Signature of Therapist**

Therapy – 3

Name:	
Age:	
Sex:	
Address:	
Religion:	
Education:	
Occupation:	
Marital status:	
Informant:	
Date of admission:	
MRD No.:	
Diagnosis:	

Therapy Attended: _____ **Session:** _____

Date: _____ **Duration (in mints):** _____

Steps of Procedure: _____

_____

_____

_____

_____

_____

_____

Summary:_____

_____

_____

Signature of Student   **Signature of Therapist**

Therapy – 4

Name:	
Age:	
Sex:	
Address:	
Religion:	
Education:	
Occupation:	
Marital status:	
Informant:	
Date of admission:	
MRD No.:	
Diagnosis:	

Therapy Attended: _____ **Session:** _____

Date: _____ **Duration (in mints):** _____

Steps of Procedure: _____

_____
_____
_____
_____
_____
_____
_____

Summary: _____

_____
_____
_____

Signature of Student   **Signature of Therapist**

Therapy – 5

Name:	
Age:	
Sex:	
Address:	
Religion:	
Education:	
Occupation:	
Marital status:	
Informant:	
Date of admission:	
MRD No.:	
Diagnosis:	

Therapy Attended: _____ **Session:** _____

Date: _____ **Duration (in mints):** _____

Steps of Procedure: _____

_____

_____

_____

_____

_____

_____

_____

Summary: _____

_____

_____

_____

Signature of Student   **Signature of Therapist**

PSYCHOMETRIC ASSESSMENT

Psychometric Assessment: A psychometric test is a scientific method used by expert to assess a patient's mental ability, personality and behaviour.

Psychometric Assessment; Observational Report – 1

Introduction:

Procedure:

Test comprise of:

Verbal (Component)	Performance

Time taken for completion:

Final impression:
- _____
- _____
- _____
- _____
- _____

Signature of Psychologist

Psychometric Assessment; Observational Report – 2

Introduction:

Procedure:

Test comprise of:

Verbal (Component)	Performance

Time taken for completion:

Final impression:

- _____
- _____
- _____
- _____
- _____

Signature of Psychologist

Psychometric Assessment; Observational Report – 3

Introduction:

Procedure:

Test comprise of:

Verbal (Component)	Performance

Time taken for completion:

Final impression:
- _____
- _____
- _____
- _____
- _____

Signature of Psychologist

Psychometric Assessment; Observational Report – 4

Introduction:

Procedure:

Test comprise of:

Verbal (Component)	Performance

Time taken for completion:

Final impression:

- _____
- _____
- _____
- _____
- _____

Signature of Psychologist

Psychometric Assessment; Observational Report – 5

Introduction:

Procedure:

Test comprise of:

Verbal (Component)	Performance

Time taken for completion:

Final impression:

- _____
- _____
- _____
- _____
- _____

Signature of Psychologist

CASE STUDY

A detailed assessment and systematic description of one patient or group of similar patients to promote a detailed understanding of their case. It helps student to understand how to assess, diagnose, treat the condition, in the case study student follow the patient from admission to discharge. Which include history, physical examination, MSC, treatment, nurses care plan, etc.

Case Study

Objectives of Case Study – 1

General Objectives:

Specific Objectives:
The specific objectives of the case study are:

Biographic Data:

1. **Health History:**

A. Demographic Data:

Name:	
Age:	
Sex:	
Address:	
Religion:	
Education:	
Occupation:	
Marital status:	
Informant:	
Date of admission:	
Date of discharge:	
MRD No.:	
Attending doctor:	
Diagnosis:	

B. Chief Complaints:

C. History of Present Illness:

D. Patient Complaints of:
-
-
-
-
-
-
-
-
-
-

E. Past Psychiatric and Medical History:
-
-
-
-
-
-
-
-
-
-

Substance Use Details:

F. Family History:

No. of family members:

Family Tree

G. Personal history:		
Perinatal history:		
Childhood history:	Primary caregiver:	
	Feeding:	
	Developmental milestones:	
	Behavior and emotional problems:	
	Illness during childhood:	
Educational history:		
Play history:		
Emotional problems during adolescence:		
Puberty:		
Dietary history:		
Occupational history:		
Marital history:		
Pre-morbid personality:		
• Family and social relationships:		
• Use of leisure time:		
• Religious beliefs:		
• Predominant mood:		
• Habits:		
• Eating pattern:		
• Elimination:		
• Sleep:		
H. Allergies:		
I. Socioeconomic status:		
J. Environmental factor:		
K. Housing pattern:		
L. Waste disposal:		

Physical Assessment

General Survey:	
Height = Weight =	cm kg
Skin:	
Head:	
Eyes:	
Eye brows:	
Eyelashes:	
Eyelids:	
Eyeballs:	
Conjunctiva:	
Pupil:	
Lens:	
Vision:	
Ears:	
External ears:	
Nose:	
External nares:	
Nostrils:	
Mouth:	
Lips:	
Tongue:	
Gums:	
Teeth:	
Neck:	
Thyroid:	
Lymph nodes:	
Cardiovascular system:	
Pulse rate:	
On Auscultation:	
Respiratory system:	
Respiratory rate:	
Gastrointestinal system:	
Appetite:	
Bowel Habits:	
Abdominal finding:	

Genitourinary system:	
Musculoskeletal system:	
Gait:	
Posture:	
Central nervous system:	
Orientation to: • Time: • Place: • Person:	
Sociological system: **Relationship:**	
Do you agree with female feticide:	
Do you treat gender equally:	
Do you give same preference to gender education equality:	
Do you condemn drug addiction:	
Do you like social gatherings:	
Do you agree with concept that one should show differences between religion/caste/creed/color	
Economic status:	
Total income per month:	
Total number of family members:	
Mental and emotional status:	
Feeling right towards others:	
Able to take decisions independently:	
Feels depressed over very often for simple reasons:	
Are you worried always without any reason:	
Spiritual aspects:	
Follows religious beliefs:	
Understands religious concepts:	
Do you get satisfaction in attending religious places:	
Vital signs:	
Temperature:	°F.
Pulse rate:	/minute
Respiratory rate:	/minute
Blood pressure:	/mm Hg

Any other observations during physical examination

Laboratory Investigations

S. No.	Test	Patient value	Normal value	Remarks
1.	Hemogram: Hemoglobin TLC MCV HCT WBC LYMPH NEUT MONO EISONO BASO PLT	gm/dL /cumm fl % /cumm % % % % % /cumm	13–18 gm/dL 4,500–11000/cumm 75–95fl 40–50% 4–10/cumm 20–25% 40–75% 01–10% 1–6% 00–01% 140–440/cumm	
2.	KFT: Urea Creatinine	mg/dL mg/dL	10–50 mg/dL 0.5–1.5 mg/dL	
3.	Electrolytes: Na^+ K^+ pH PO_2	mmol/L mmol/L mm Hg	135–145 mmol/L 3.5–5.0 mmol/L 7.35–7.45 85–95 mm Hg	
4.	Serum Chemistry: Uric acid Calcium Blood glucose Random Fasting Post prandial	mg/dL mg/dL mg/dL ....mg/dL ....mg/dL	2.5–8 mg/dL 8.6–10.2 mg/dL 70 –140 mg/dL 60–110 mg/dL 65–140 mg/dL	
5.	LFT: Bilirubin AST ALT ALP Albumin	mg/dL U/L U/mL UL g/dL	0.3–1.0 mg/dL 15–30 U/L 8–35 U/mL 50–120 UL 3.5–5.5 g/dL	

Mental Status Examination (MSE)

I. General Appearance and Behavior (GAAB):
  a. Facial expression (e.g., anxiety, pleasure, confidence, blunted, pleasant): _____
  b. Posture (stooped, stiff, guarded, normal): _____
  c. Mannerisms (stereotype, negativism, tics, normal): _____
  d. Eye to eye contact (maintained or not): _____
  e. Rapport (built easily or not built or built with difficulty): _____
  f. Consciousness (conscious or drowsy or unconscious): _____
  g. Behavior (includes social behavior, e.g., overfriendly, disinherited, preoccupied, aggressive, normal): _____
  h. Dressing and grooming – well-dressed/appropriate/inappropriate (to season and situation)/neat and tidy/dirty:
  i. Physical features: Looks of one's age/look older/younger than his or her age/underweight/overweight/physical deformity: _____

II. Psychomotor Activity:
Increased/decreased/compulsive/echopraxia/stereotypy/negativism/automatic obedience:
_____

III. Speech: One sample of speech (verbatim in 2 or 3 sentences):
   a. Coherence—Coherent/incoherent: _____
   b. Relevance (answer the questions appropriately)—Relevant/irrelevant: _____
   c. Volume (soft, loud or normal): _____
   d. Tone (high pitch, low pitch, or normal/monotonous): _____
   e. Manner—Excessive formal/relaxed/inappropriately familiar: _____
   f. Reaction time (time taken to answer the question)—Increased, decreased or normal: _____
   _____

IV. Thought:
   a. Form of thought/formal thought disorder—not understandable/normal/circumstantiality/tangentiality/neologism/word salad/preservation/ambivalence: _____
   b. Stream of thought/flow of thought—pressure of speech/flight of ideas/thought retardation/mutism/aphonia/thought block/Clang association: _____
   c. Content of thought
      i. Delusions (specify type and give example)—Persecutory/delusion of reference/delusions of influence or passivity/hypochondriacal delusions/delusions of grandeur/nihilistic—Derealization/depersonalization/delusions of infidelity: _____
      ii. Obsession: _____
      iii. Phobia: _____
      iv. Pre-occupation: _____
      v. Fantasy—Creative/day dreaming: _____

V. Mood (subjective) and Affect (objective):
   a. Appropriate/inappropriate (Relevance to situation and thought congruent): _____
   b. Pleasurable affect—Euphoria/Elation/Exaltation/Ecstasy: _____
   c. Unpleasurable affect—Grief/mourning/depression: _____
   d. Other affects—Anxiety/fear/panic/free floating anxiety/apathy/aggression/moods swing/emotional liability:
   _____

VI. Disorders Perception: _____
   a. Illusion: _____
   b. Hallucinations (specify type and give example)—Auditory/visual/olfactory/gustatory/tactile: _____
   _____
   c. Others—Hypnologic/hypnopombic/lilliputian/kinesthetic/macropsia/micropsia: _____
   _____

VII. Cognitive Functions:
   a. Attention and concentration:
      - Method of testing (Asking to list the months of the year forward and backward): _____
      - Serial subtractions (100-7): _____
   b. Memory:
      a. Immediate (Teach an address and after 5 minutes. Asking for recall): _____
      b. Recent memory – 24 hrs. recall: _____
      c. Remote: Asking for dates of birth or events which are occurred long back: _____
   c. Orientation:
      a. Time—Approximately without looking at the watch, what time is it? _____
      b. Place—Where he/she is now? _____
      c. Person—Who has accompanied him or her? _____
   d. Abstraction: Give a proverb and ask the inner meaning (e.g., feathers of a bird flock together/rolling stones gather no mass): _____
   e. Intelligence and general information: Test by carry over sums/similarities and differences/and general information/digit score test: _____

f. Judgment:
      - Personal (future plans): _____
      - Social (perception of the society): _____
      - Test (present a situation and ask their response to the situation): _____
        _____

   g. Insight:
      a. Complete denial of illness: _____
      b. Slight awareness of being sick: _____
      c. Awareness of being sick attribute it to external/physical factor: _____
      d. Awareness of being sick, but due to something unknown in himself: _____
      e. Intellectual insight: _____
      f. True emotional insight: _____

VIII. General Observations:
   a. Sleep
      i. Insomnia—temporary/persistent: _____
      ii. Hypersomnia—temporary/persistent: _____
      iii. Non-organic sleep—wake cycle disturbance: _____
      iv. EMA—Early Morning Awakening: _____
   b. Episodic disturbances—Epilepsy/hysterical/impulsive behavior/aggressive behavior/destructive behavior:
      _____

IX. Summary and Clinical Diagnosis evaluation: After a long history of psychiatric illness the patient was diagnosed as ' '.

Definition, Cause and Psychopathology of Patients Disease

Etiology

  i. **Biological theories:**

  ii. **Biochemical theories:**

 iii. **Genetic theories:**

 iv. **Psychodynamic theories:**

  v. **Developmental theories:**

 vi. **Family theories:**

vii. **Social factors:**

Clinical Types:

Psychopathology:

Signs and Symptoms

According to book	According to patient

Diagnostic Evaluation

According to book	Patient picture

Treatment Modalities

Book picture	Patient picture

Nursing Management

Effective communication techniques:

Maintain safety:

Providing structure:

Ways to reduce or minimize psychosis:

Summary of patient's daily progress report in hospital

Date	Temperature	Pulse	Respiration	Blood pressure	Summary
-	°F	b/min	/min	/mm Hg	
-	°F	b/min	/min	/mm Hg	
-	°F	b/min	/min	/mm Hg	
-	°F	b/min	/min	/mm Hg	

Nursing Diagnosis

-
-
-
-
-
-

Assessment	Nursing diagnosis	Planning/Goal	Intervention	Rationale	Evaluation

Assessment	Nursing diagnosis	Planning/Goal	Intervention	Rationale	Evaluation

Assessment	Nursing diagnosis	Planning/Goal	Intervention	Rationale	Evaluation

Assessment	Nursing diagnosis	Planning/Goal	Intervention	Rationale	Evaluation

Discharge Teaching:

- **Diet:** _____
- _____
- _____
- _____
- _____
- _____
- _____

Conclusion and Summary of Case Study:

Clinical Evaluation Remarks

Case study is the comprehensive study of one selected patient and comparative study with books. During my case study, I learned the following things.

1. About the disease:

2. About the patients:

3. About nursing care:

4. About documentation:

References

Objectives of Case Study – 2

General Objectives:

Specific Objectives:
The specific objectives of the case study are:

Biographic Data:
1. **Health History:**
A. Demographic Data:

Name:	
Age:	
Sex:	
Address:	
Religion:	
Education:	
Occupation:	
Marital status:	
Informant:	
Date of admission:	
Date of discharge:	
MRD No.:	
Attending doctor:	
Diagnosis:	

B. Chief Complaints:

C. History of Present Illness:

D. Patient Complaints of:
-
-
-
-
-
-
-
-
-
-

E. Past Psychiatric and Medical History:
-
-
-
-
-
-
-
-
-

Substance Use Details:

F. Family History:

No. of family members:

Family Tree

G. Personal history:		
Perinatal history:		
Childhood history:	Primary caregiver:	
	Feeding:	
	Developmental milestones:	
	Behavior and emotional problems:	
	Illness during childhood:	
Educational history:		
Play history:		
Emotional problems during adolescence:		
Puberty:		
Dietary history:		
Occupational history:		
Marital history:		
Pre-morbid personality:		
• Family and social relationships:		
• Use of leisure time:		
• Religious beliefs:		
• Predominant mood:		
• Habits:		
• Eating pattern:		
• Elimination:		
• Sleep:		
H. Allergies:		
I. Socioeconomic status:		
J. Environmental factor:		
K. Housing pattern:		
L. Waste disposal:		

Physical Assessment

General Survey:	
Height =	cm
Weight =	kg
Skin:	
Head:	
Eyes:	
Eye brows:	
Eyelashes:	
Eyelids:	
Eyeballs:	
Conjunctiva:	
Pupil:	
Lens:	
Vision:	
Ears:	
External ears:	
Nose:	
External nares:	
Nostrils:	
Mouth:	
LIPS:	
Tongue:	
Gums:	
Teeth:	
Neck:	
Thyroid:	
Lymph nodes:	
Cardiovascular system:	
Pulse rate:	
On Auscultation:	
Respiratory system:	
Respiratory rate:	
Gastrointestinal system:	
Appetite:	
Bowel Habits:	
Abdominal finding:	

Genitourinary system:	
Musculoskeletal system:	
Gait:	
Posture:	
Central nervous system:	
Orientation to: • Time: • Place: • Person:	
Sociological system: **Relationship:**	
Do you agree with female feticide:	
Do you treat gender equally:	
Do you give same preference to gender education equality:	
Do you condemn drug addiction:	
Do you like social gatherings:	
Do you agree with concept that one should show differences between religion/caste/creed/color	
Economic status:	
Total income per month:	
Total number of family members:	
Mental and emotional status:	
Feeling right towards others:	
Able to take decisions independently:	
Feels depressed over very often for simple reasons:	
Are you worried always without any reason:	
Spiritual aspects:	
Follows religious beliefs:	
Understands religious concepts:	
Do you get satisfaction in attending religious places:	
Vital signs:	
Temperature:	°F.
Pulse rate:	/minute
Respiratory rate:	/minute
Blood pressure:	/mm Hg

Any other observations during physical examination

Laboratory Investigations

S. No.	Test	Patient value	Normal value	Remarks
1.	Hemogram: Hemoglobin TLC MCV HCT WBC LYMPH NEUT MONO EISONO BASO PLT	gm/dL /cumm fl % /cumm % % % % % /cumm	13–18 gm/dL 4,500–11000/cumm 75–95fl 40–50% 4–10/cumm 20–25% 40–75% 01–10% 1–6% 00–01% 140–440/cumm	
2.	KFT: Urea Creatinine	mg/dL mg/dL	10–50 mg/dL 0.5–1.5 mg/dL	
3.	Electrolytes: Na⁺ K⁺ pH PO$_2$	mmol/L mmol/L mm Hg	135–145 mmol/L 3.5–5.0 mmol/L 7.35–7.45 85–95 mm Hg	
4.	Serum Chemistry: Uric acid Calcium Blood glucose Random Fasting Post prandial	mg/dL mg/dL mg/dL ....mg/dL ....mg/dL	2.5–8 mg/dL 8.6–10.2 mg/dL 70–140 mg/dL 60–110 mg/dL 65–140 mg/dL	
5.	LFT: Bilirubin AST ALT ALP Albumin	mg/dL U/L U/mL UL g/dL	0.3–1.0 mg/dL 15–30 U/L 8–35 U/mL 50–120 UL 3.5–5.5 g/dL	

Mental Status Examination (MSE)

I. General Appearance and Behavior (GAAB):
   a. Facial expression (e.g., anxiety, pleasure, confidence, blunted, pleasant): _____
   b. Posture (stooped, stiff, guarded, normal): _____
   c. Mannerisms (stereotype, negativism, tics, normal): _____
   d. Eye to eye contact (maintained or not): _____
   e. Rapport (built easily or not built or built with difficulty): _____
   f. Consciousness (conscious or drowsy or unconscious): _____
   g. Behavior (includes social behavior, e.g., overfriendly, disinherited, preoccupied, aggressive, normal): _____
   h. Dressing and grooming – well-dressed/appropriate/inappropriate (to season and situation)/neat and tidy/dirty: _____
   i. Physical features: Looks of one's age/look older/younger than his or her age/underweight/overweight/physical deformity: _____

II. Psychomotor Activity:
Increased/decreased/compulsive/echopraxia/stereotypy/negativism/automatic obedience: _____

III. Speech: One sample of speech (verbatim in 2 or 3 sentences):
   a. Coherence—Coherent/incoherent: _____
   b. Relevance (answer the questions appropriately)—Relevant/irrelevant: _____
   c. Volume (soft, loud or normal): _____
   d. Tone (high pitch, low pitch, or normal/monotonous): _____
   e. Manner—Excessive formal/relaxed/inappropriately familiar: _____
   f. Reaction time (time taken to answer the question)—Increased, decreased or normal: _____

IV. Thought:
   a. Form of thought/formal thought disorder—not understandable/normal/circumstantiality/tangentiality/neologism/word salad/preservation/ambivalence: _____
   b. Stream of thought/flow of thought—pressure of speech/flight of ideas/thought retardation/mutism/aphonia/thought block/Clang association: _____
   c. Content of thought
      i. Delusions (specify type and give example)—Persecutory/delusion of reference/delusions of influence or passivity/hypochondriacal delusions/delusions of grandeur/nihilistic—Derealization/depersonalization/delusions of infidelity: _____
      ii. Obsession: _____
      iii. Phobia: _____
      iv. Pre-occupation: _____
      v. Fantasy—Creative/day dreaming: _____

V. Mood (subjective) and Affect (objective):
   a. Appropriate/inappropriate (Relevance to situation and thought congruent): _____
   b. Pleasurable affect—Euphoria/Elation/Exaltation/Ecstasy: _____
   c. Unpleasurable affect—Grief/mourning/depression: _____
   d. Other affects—Anxiety/fear/panic/free floating anxiety/apathy/aggression/moods swing/emotional liability: _____

VI. Disorders Perception: _____
   a. Illusion: _____
   b. Hallucinations (specify type and give example)—Auditory/visual/olfactory/gustatory/tactile: _____
   c. Others—Hypnologic/hypnopombic/lilliputian/kinesthetic/macropsia/micropsia: _____

VII. Cognitive Functions:
   a. Attention and concentration:
      - Method of testing (Asking to list the months of the year forward and backward): _____
      - Serial subtractions (100-7): _____
   b. Memory:
      a. Immediate (Teach an address and after 5 minutes. Asking for recall): _____
      b. Recent memory – 24 hrs. recall: _____
      c. Remote: Asking for dates of birth or events which are occurred long back: _____
   c. Orientation:
      a. Time—Approximately without looking at the watch, what time is it? _____
      b. Place—Where he/she is now? _____
      c. Person—Who has accompanied him or her? _____
   d. Abstraction: Give a proverb and ask the inner meaning (e.g., feathers of a bird flock together/rolling stones gather no mass): _____
   e. Intelligence and general information: Test by carry over sums/similarities and differences/and general information/digit score test: _____

f. Judgment:
   - Personal (future plans): _____
   - Social (perception of the society): _____
   - Test (present a situation and ask their response to the situation): _____
   _____

g. Insight:
   a. Complete denial of illness: _____
   b. Slight awareness of being sick: _____
   c. Awareness of being sick attribute it to external/physical factor: _____
   d. Awareness of being sick, but due to something unknown in himself: _____
   e. Intellectual insight: _____
   f. True emotional insight: _____

VIII. General Observations:
   a. Sleep:
      i. Insomnia—temporary/persistent: _____
      ii. Hypersomnia—temporary/persistent: _____
      iii. Non-organic sleep—wake cycle disturbance: _____
      iv. EMA—Early Morning Awakening: _____
   b. Episodic disturbances—Epilepsy/hysterical/impulsive behavior/aggressive behavior/destructive behavior:
   _____

IX. Summary and Clinical Diagnosis evaluation: After a long history of psychiatric illness the patient was diagnosed as ' '.

Definition, Cause and Psychopathology of Patients Disease

Etiology

i. Biological theories:

ii. Biochemical theories:

iii. Genetic theories:

iv. Psychodynamic theories:

v. Developmental theories:

vi. Family theories:

vii. Social factors:

Clinical Types:

Psychopathology:

Signs and Symptoms

According to book	According to patient

Diagnostic Evaluation

According to book	Patient picture

Treatment Modalities

Book picture	Patient picture

Nursing Management

Effective communication techniques:

Maintain safety:

Providing structure:

Ways to reduce or minimize psychosis:

Summary of patient's daily progress report in hospital

Date	Temperature	Pulse	Respiration	Blood pressure	Summary
-	°F	b/min	/min	/mm Hg	
-	°F	b/min	/min	/mm Hg	
-	°F	b/min	/min	/mm Hg	
-	°F	b/min	/min	/mm Hg	

Nursing Diagnosis

-
-
-
-
-
-

Assessment	Nursing diagnosis	Planning/Goal	Intervention	Rationale	Evaluation

Assessment	Nursing diagnosis	Planning/Goal	Intervention	Rationale	Evaluation

Assessment	Nursing diagnosis	Planning/Goal	Intervention	Rationale	Evaluation

Assessment	Nursing diagnosis	Planning/Goal	Intervention	Rationale	Evaluation

Discharge Teaching:

- Diet: _____
- _____
- _____
- _____
- _____
- _____
- _____

Conclusion and Summary of Case Study:

Clinical Evaluation Remarks

Case study is the comprehensive study of one selected patient and comparative study with books. During my case study, I learned the following things.

1. **About the disease:**

2. **About the patients:**

3. **About nursing care:**

4. **About documentation:**

References

Objectives of Case Study – 3

General Objectives:

Specific Objectives:
The specific objectives of the case study are:

Biographic Data:
1. **Health History**:
A. Demographic Data:

Name:	
Age:	
Sex:	
Address:	
Religion:	
Education:	
Occupation:	
Marital status:	
Informant:	
Date of admission:	
Date of discharge:	
MRD No.:	
Attending doctor:	
Diagnosis:	

B. Chief Complaints:

C. History of Present Illness:

D. Patient Complaints of:
-
-
-
-
-
-
-
-
-
-

E. Past Psychiatric and Medical History:
-
-
-
-
-
-
-
-
-
-

Substance Use Details:

F. Family History:

No. of family members:

Family Tree

G. Personal history:			
Perinatal history:			
Childhood history:	Primary caregiver:		
	Feeding:		
	Developmental milestones:		
	Behavior and emotional problems:		
	Illness during childhood:		
Educational history:			
Play history:			
Emotional problems during adolescence:			
Puberty:			
Dietary history:			
Occupational history:			
Marital history:			
Pre-morbid personality:			
• Family and social relationships:			
• Use of leisure time:			
• Religious beliefs:			
• Predominant mood:			
• Habits:			
• Eating pattern:			
• Elimination:			
• Sleep:			
H. Allergies:			
I. Socioeconomic status:			
J. Environmental factor:			
K. Housing pattern:			
L. Waste disposal:			

Physical Assessment

General Survey:	
Height = **Weight =**	cm kg
Skin:	
Head:	
Eyes:	
Eye brows:	
Eyelashes:	
Eyelids:	
Eyeballs:	
Conjunctiva:	
Pupil:	
Lens:	
Vision:	
Ears:	
External ears:	
Nose:	
External nares:	
Nostrils:	
Mouth:	
LIPS:	
Tongue:	
Gums:	
Teeth:	
Neck:	
Thyroid:	
Lymph nodes:	
Cardiovascular system:	
Pulse rate:	
On Auscultation:	
Respiratory system:	
Respiratory rate:	
Gastrointestinal system:	
Appetite:	
Bowel Habits:	
Abdominal finding:	

Genitourinary system:	
Musculoskeletal system:	
Gait:	
Posture:	
Central nervous system:	
Orientation to: • Time: • Place: • Person:	
Sociological system: **Relationship:**	
Do you agree with female feticide:	
Do you treat gender equally:	
Do you give same preference to gender education equality:	
Do you condemn drug addiction:	
Do you like social gatherings:	
Do you agree with concept that one should show differences between religion/caste/creed/color	
Economic status:	
Total income per month:	
Total number of family members:	
Mental and emotional status:	
Feeling right towards others:	
Able to take decisions independently:	
Feels depressed over very often for simple reasons:	
Are you worried always without any reason:	
Spiritual aspects:	
Follows religious beliefs:	
Understands religious concepts:	
Do you get satisfaction in attending religious places:	
Vital signs:	
Temperature:	°F.
Pulse rate:	/minute
Respiratory rate:	/minute
Blood pressure:	/mm Hg

Any other observations during physical examination

Laboratory Investigations

S. No.	Test	Patient value	Normal value	Remarks
1.	Hemogram: Hemoglobin TLC MCV HCT WBC LYMPH NEUT MONO EISONO BASO PLT	gm/dL /cumm fl % /cumm % % % % % /cumm	13–18 gm/dL 4,500–11000/cumm 75–95fl 40–50% 4–10/cumm 20–25% 40–75% 01–10% 1–6% 00–01% 140–440/cumm	
2.	KFT: Urea Creatinine	mg/dL mg/dL	10–50 mg/dL 0.5–1.5 mg/dL	
3.	Electrolytes: Na$^+$ K$^+$ pH PO$_2$	mmol/L mmol/L mm Hg	135–145 mmol/L 3.5–5.0 mmol/L 7.35–7.45 85–95 mm Hg	
4.	Serum Chemistry: Uric acid Calcium Blood glucose Random Fasting Post prandial	mg/dL mg/dL mg/dL ....mg/dL ....mg/dL	2.5–8 mg/dL 8.6–10.2 mg/dL 70 –140 mg/dL 60–110 mg/dL 65–140 mg/dL	
5.	LFT: Bilirubin AST ALT ALP Albumin	mg/dL U/L U/mL UL g/dL	0.3–1.0 mg/dL 15–30 U/L 8–35 U/mL 50–120 UL 3.5–5.5 g/dL	

Mental Status Examination (MSE)

I. General Appearance and Behavior (GAAB):
   a. Facial expression (e.g., anxiety, pleasure, confidence, blunted, pleasant): _____
   b. Posture (stooped, stiff, guarded, normal): _____
   c. Mannerisms (stereotype, negativism, tics, normal): _____
   d. Eye to eye contact (maintained or not): _____
   e. Rapport (built easily or not built or built with difficulty): _____
   f. Consciousness (conscious or drowsy or unconscious): _____
   g. Behavior (includes social behavior, e.g., overfriendly, disinherited, preoccupied, aggressive, normal): _____
   h. Dressing and grooming – well-dressed/appropriate/inappropriate (to season and situation)/neat and tidy/dirty: _____
   i. Physical features: Looks of one's age/look older/younger than his or her age/underweight/overweight/physical deformity: _____

II. Psychomotor Activity:
Increased/decreased/compulsive/echopraxia/stereotypy/negativism/automatic obedience: _____

III. Speech: One sample of speech (verbatim in 2 or 3 sentences):
a. Coherence—Coherent/incoherent: _____
b. Relevance (answer the questions appropriately)—Relevant/irrelevant: _____
c. Volume (soft, loud or normal): _____
d. Tone (high pitch, low pitch, or normal/monotonous): _____
e. Manner—Excessive formal/relaxed/inappropriately familiar: _____
f. Reaction time (time taken to answer the question)—Increased, decreased or normal: _____

IV. Thought:
a. Form of thought/formal thought disorder—not understandable/normal/circumstantiality/tangentiality/neologism/word salad/preservation/ambivalence: _____
b. Stream of thought/flow of thought—pressure of speech/flight of ideas/thought retardation/mutism/aphonia/thought block/Clang association: _____
c. Content of thought
   i. Delusions (specify type and give example)—Persecutory/delusion of reference/delusions of influence or passivity/hypochondriacal delusions/delusions of grandeur/nihilistic—Derealization/depersonalization/delusions of infidelity: _____
   ii. Obsession: _____
   iii. Phobia: _____
   iv. Pre-occupation: _____
   v. Fantasy—Creative/day dreaming: _____

V. Mood (subjective) and Affect (objective):
a. Appropriate/inappropriate (Relevance to situation and thought congruent): _____
b. Pleasurable affect—Euphoria/Elation/Exaltation/Ecstasy: _____
c. Unpleasurable affect—Grief/mourning/depression: _____
d. Other affects—Anxiety/fear/panic/free floating anxiety/apathy/aggression/moods swing/emotional liability: _____

VI. Disorders Perception: _____
a. Illusion: _____
b. Hallucinations (specify type and give example)—Auditory/visual/olfactory/gustatory/tactile: _____
c. Others—Hypnologic/hypnopombic/lilliputian/kinesthetic/macropsia/micropsia: _____

VII. Cognitive Functions:
a. Attention and concentration:
   - Method of testing (Asking to list the months of the year forward and backward): _____
   - Serial subtractions (100-7): _____
b. Memory:
   a. Immediate (Teach an address and after 5 minutes. Asking for recall): _____
   b. Recent memory – 24 hrs. recall: _____
   c. Remote: Asking for dates of birth or events which are occurred long back: _____
c. Orientation:
   a. Time—Approximately without looking at the watch, what time is it? _____
   b. Place—Where he/she is now? _____
   c. Person—Who has accompanied him or her? _____
d. Abstraction: Give a proverb and ask the inner meaning (e.g., feathers of a bird flock together/rolling stones gather no mass): _____
e. Intelligence and general information: Test by carry over sums/similarities and differences/and general information/digit score test: _____

f. Judgment:
   - Personal (future plans): _____
   - Social (perception of the society): _____
   - Test (present a situation and ask their response to the situation): _____
   _____

g. Insight:
   a. Complete denial of illness: _____
   b. Slight awareness of being sick: _____
   c. Awareness of being sick attribute it to external/physical factor: _____
   d. Awareness of being sick, but due to something unknown in himself: _____
   e. Intellectual insight: _____
   f. True emotional insight: _____

VIII. General Observations:
   a. Sleep:
      i. Insomnia—temporary/persistent: _____
      ii. Hypersomnia—temporary/persistent: _____
      iii. Non-organic sleep—wake cycle disturbance: _____
      iv. EMA—Early Morning Awakening: _____
   b. Episodic disturbances—Epilepsy/hysterical/impulsive behavior/aggressive behavior/destructive behavior:
   _____

IX. Summary and Clinical Diagnosis evaluation: After a long history of psychiatric illness the patient was diagnosed as ' '.

Definition, Cause and Psychopathology of Patients Disease

Etiology

   i. **Biological theories:**

  ii. **Biochemical theories:**

 iii. **Genetic theories:**

  iv. **Psychodynamic theories:**

   v. **Developmental theories:**

  vi. **Family theories:**

 vii. **Social factors:**

Clinical Types:

Psychopathology:

Signs and Symptoms

According to book	According to patient

Diagnostic Evaluation

According to book	Patient picture

Treatment Modalities

Book picture	Patient picture

Nursing Management

Effective communication techniques:

Maintain safety:

Providing structure:

Ways to reduce or minimize psychosis:

Summary of patient's daily progress report in hospital

Date	Temperature	Pulse	Respiration	Blood pressure	Summary
-	°F	b/min	/min	/mm Hg	
-	°F	b/min	/min	/mm Hg	
-	°F	b/min	/min	/mm Hg	
-	°F	b/min	/min	/mm Hg	

Nursing Diagnosis

-
-
-
-
-
-

Assessment	Nursing diagnosis	Planning/Goal	Intervention	Rationale	Evaluation

Assessment	Nursing diagnosis	Planning/Goal	Intervention	Rationale	Evaluation

Assessment	Nursing diagnosis	Planning/Goal	Intervention	Rationale	Evaluation

Assessment	Nursing diagnosis	Planning/Goal	Intervention	Rationale	Evaluation

Discharge Teaching:

- **Diet:** _____
- _____
- _____
- _____
- _____
- _____
- _____

Conclusion and Summary of Case Study:

Clinical Evaluation Remarks

Case study is the comprehensive study of one selected patient and comparative study with books. During my case study, I learned the following things.

1. About the disease:

2. About the patients:

3. About nursing care:

4. About documentation:

References

COMMUNITY MENTAL HEALTH NURSING: CASE WORK

COMMUNITY MENTAL HEALTH NURSING

Guidelines for Community Mental Health Nursing
1. Identification of community leader and resource person.
2. Conduct community health survey.
3. Mental health assessment.
4. Mental status examination.
5. Physical examination.
6. Incidental health teaching.
7. Teaching parenting skills and child development to new parents (marriage counseling).
8. Teaching drug hazards to the school children in various age groups.
9. Teaching techniques of stress management to the individuals who are in need (JPMR).
10. Teaching ways how to coup up with pain full situation.
11. Providing education and support to un-employed widows, new retires and women entering in the menopausal group.
12. Ongoing assessment of individual at high risk (exposed to continuous stress).
13. Provision of care for individuals in whom mentally ill symptoms are visible.
14. Referral of individual to hospital in whom symptoms are visible and not treated at community level.
15. Prevention of relapses if a person is on anti-psychotic drugs by educating him not to discontinue the medication.

Objectives to be Filled
1. Discuss the changing focus of care in the field of mental health in the community.
2. Discuss the concept of care in the field of mental illness in the community.
3. Discuss the concept of primary, secondary and tertiary prevention within the community.
4. Identify the population at risk for mental illness with in the community.
5. Discuss nursing intervention in primary, secondary and tertiary prevention of mental illness within the community.
6. Relate historical, epidemiological factors associated with caring for the seriously mentally ill and homeless mentally ill within the community.
7. Identify the alternative for the care of the seriously mentally ill and homeless mentally ill patients within the community.
8. Apply steps of nursing process for the care of serious mentally ill and homeless mentally ill patients within the community.

Data from Community Leader
1. Knowledge about the village: _____
2. Achievements if any: _____
3. Number of schools in total: _____
   3.1 Primary: _____
   3.2 Secondary: _____
   3.3 Higher secondary: _____
4. Health facilities: _____
5. Environment sanitation data: _____
   5.1 Water supply: _____
   5.2 Excreta disposal: _____
   5.3 Waste disposal: _____

6. **Communication facilities:** _____
    6.1 **Transport:** _____
    6.2 **STD's:** _____
    6.3 **Telegraph office:** _____
    6.4 **Post office:** _____
    6.5 **Bank:** _____
    6.6 **Availability of markets:** _____
    6.7 **Dealing with emergencies:** _____
    6.8 **Recreation facilities:** _____

Future plans for further development:

Community Case Work – 1

Mental Health Assessment:

1. **Geographical Assessment:**
    - Name of the place/area: _____
    - Rural/Urban: _____
    - Name of the PHC/Sub-center: _____
2. **Family Identification Information:**
    - Name of the head of the family: _____
    - Type of the family: _____
    - Religion: _____
    - Caste: _____
    - Address: _____
3. **Family Characteristics and Health Status of the Family Members:**

S. No.	Name of the family member	Age	Sex	Relationship with the head of the family	Education and occupation	Health (any stressor)
1.						
2.						
3.						
4.						
5.						
6.						

4. **Housing Condition:**
    - Type of house: _____
    - No. of rooms: _____
    - Ventilation: _____
    - Lighting: _____
    - Water supply: _____
    - Kitchen: _____
    - Smoke outlet: _____
    - Bath room: _____
    - Latrine: _____
    - Drainage: _____
    - Refuse disposal: _____
    - Cattle shed: _____
    - Utilization of health services: _____

5. **Socioeconomic Status:**
    - House: _____
    - Land: _____
    - Income of the family per month: _____
    - Facilities at home: _____
6. **Transport and Communication:**
    - Type of road: _____
    - Transport facilities: _____
    - Communication facilities: _____
7. **Nutritional Pattern:**
    - Food habits: _____
    _____
    - Assessment of support system: _____
    _____
    - Relationship with neighbors: _____
    - Relationship with relatives: _____
8. **Assessment of Risk Factors for Mental Health:**

S. No.	Name of family member	Present health status	Any chronic disease	Specify any stressor
1.				
2.				
3.				

- Family history of mental illness: _____
- Use of leisure: _____
- Recreational activities/relaxation activities: _____
_____
- Describe cultural practices related to health: _____
_____
- Describe religious practices/festivals: _____
_____
- Interpersonal relationship among family members: _____
_____
- Any addictions: _____
- Vital occurrence during last one year: _____
- History of past illness: _____

- **Physical handicap:** _____
- **Mental retardation:** _____
- **History of epilepsy/suicide:** _____
- **Knowledge and attitude of family about mental health and illness:** _____

_____

Summary of family visit:

Signature of Student Nurse   **Signature of Supervisor**

Community Case Work – 2

Mental Health Assessment:

1. **Geographical Assessment:**
   - Name of the place/area: _____
   - Rural/Urban: _____
   - Name of the PHC/Sub-center: _____

2. **Family Identification Information:**
   - Name of the head of the family: _____
   - Type of the family: _____
   - Religion: _____
   - Caste: _____
   - Address: _____

3. **Family Characteristics and Health Status of the Family Members:**

S. No.	Name of the family member	Age	Sex	Relationship with the head of the family	Education and occupation	Health (any stressor)
1.						
2.						
3.						
4.						
5.						
6.						

4. **Housing Condition:**
   - Type of house: _____
   - No. of rooms: _____
   - Ventilation: _____
   - Lighting: _____
   - Water supply: _____
   - Kitchen: _____
   - Smoke outlet: _____
   - Bath room: _____
   - Latrine: _____
   - Drainage: _____
   - Refuse disposal: _____
   - Cattle shed: _____
   - Utilization of health services: _____

5. **Socioeconomic Status:**
   - House: _____
   - Land: _____
   - Income of the family per month: _____
   - Facilities at home: _____

6. **Transport and Communication:**
   - Type of road: _____
   - Transport facilities: _____
   - Communication facilities: _____

7. **Nutritional Pattern:**
   - Food habits: _____
   - Assessment of support system: _____
   - Relationship with neighbors: _____
   - Relationship with relatives: _____

8. **Assessment of Risk Factors for Mental Health:**

S. No.	Name of family member	Present health status	Any chronic disease	Specify any stressor
1.				
2.				
3.				

- Family history of mental illness: _____
- Use of leisure: _____
- Recreational activities/relaxation activities: _____
- Describe cultural practices related to health: _____
- Describe religious practices/festivals: _____
- Interpersonal relationship among family members: _____
- Any addictions: _____
- Vital occurrence during last one year: _____
- History of past illness: _____

- **Physical handicap:** _____
- **Mental retardation:** _____
- **History of epilepsy/suicide:** _____
- **Knowledge and attitude of family about mental health and illness:** _____
_____

Summary of family visit:

Signature of Student Nurse   **Signature of Supervisor**

Community Case Work – 3

Mental Health Assessment:

1. **Geographical Assessment:**
   - Name of the place/area: _____
   - Rural/Urban: _____
   - Name of the PHC/Sub-center: _____

2. **Family Identification Information:**
   - Name of the head of the family: _____
   - Type of the family: _____
   - Religion: _____
   - Caste: _____
   - Address: _____

3. **Family Characteristics and Health Status of the Family Members:**

S. No.	Name of the family member	Age	Sex	Relationship with the head of the family	Education and occupation	Health (any stressor)
1.						
2.						
3.						
4.						
5.						
6.						

4. **Housing Condition:**
   - Type of house: _____
   - No. of rooms: _____
   - Ventilation: _____
   - Lighting: _____
   - Water supply: _____
   - Kitchen: _____
   - Smoke outlet: _____
   - Bath room: _____
   - Latrine: _____
   - Drainage: _____
   - Refuse disposal: _____
   - Cattle shed: _____
   - Utilization of health services: _____

5. **Socioeconomic Status:**
   - House: _____
   - Land: _____
   - Income of the family per month: _____
   - Facilities at home: _____

6. **Transport and Communication:**
   - Type of road: _____
   - Transport facilities: _____
   - Communication facilities: _____

7. **Nutritional Pattern:**
   - Food habits: _____
   - Assessment of support system: _____
   - Relationship with neighbors: _____
   - Relationship with relatives: _____

8. **Assessment of Risk Factors for Mental Health:**

S. No.	Name of family member	Present health status	Any chronic disease	Specify any stressor
1.				
2.				
3.				

- Family history of mental illness: _____
- Use of leisure: _____
- Recreational activities/relaxation activities: _____
- Describe cultural practices related to health: _____
- Describe religious practices/festivals: _____
- Interpersonal relationship among family members: _____
- Any addictions: _____
- Vital occurrence during last one year: _____
- History of past illness: _____

- **Physical handicap:** _____
- **Mental retardation:** _____
- **History of epilepsy/suicide:** _____
- **Knowledge and attitude of family about mental health and illness:** _____
_____

Summary of family visit:

Signature of Student Nurse   **Signature of Supervisor**

Community Case Work – 4

Mental Health Assessment:

1. **Geographical Assessment:**
    - Name of the place/area: _____
    - Rural/Urban: _____
    - Name of the PHC/Sub-center: _____

2. **Family Identification Information:**
    - Name of the head of the family: _____
    - Type of the family: _____
    - Religion: _____
    - Caste: _____
    - Address: _____

3. **Family Characteristics and Health Status of the Family Members:**

S. No.	Name of the family member	Age	Sex	Relationship with the head of the family	Education and occupation	Health (any stressor)
1.						
2.						
3.						
4.						
5.						
6.						

4. **Housing Condition:**
    - Type of house: _____
    - No. of rooms: _____
    - Ventilation: _____
    - Lighting: _____
    - Water supply: _____
    - Kitchen: _____
    - Smoke outlet: _____
    - Bath room: _____
    - Latrine: _____
    - Drainage: _____
    - Refuse disposal: _____
    - Cattle shed: _____
    - Utilization of health services: _____

5. **Socioeconomic Status:**
    - House: _____
    - Land: _____
    - Income of the family per month: _____
    - Facilities at home: _____
6. **Transport and Communication:**
    - Type of road: _____
    - Transport facilities: _____
    - Communication facilities: _____
7. **Nutritional Pattern:**
    - Food habits: _____
    - Assessment of support system: _____
    - Relationship with neighbors: _____
    - Relationship with relatives: _____
8. **Assessment of Risk Factors for Mental Health:**

S. No.	Name of family member	Present health status	Any chronic disease	Specify any stressor
1.				
2.				
3.				

- Family history of mental illness: _____
- Use of leisure: _____
- Recreational activities/relaxation activities: _____
- Describe cultural practices related to health: _____
- Describe religious practices/festivals: _____
- Interpersonal relationship among family members: _____
- Any addictions: _____
- Vital occurrence during last one year: _____
- History of past illness: _____

- **Physical handicap:** _____
- **Mental retardation:** _____
- **History of epilepsy/suicide:** _____
- **Knowledge and attitude of family about mental health and illness:** _____

Summary of family visit:

Signature of Student Nurse   **Signature of Supervisor**

Community Case Work – 5

Mental Health Assessment:

1. **Geographical Assessment:**
    - Name of the place/area: _____
    - Rural/Urban: _____
    - Name of the PHC/Sub-center: _____

2. **Family Identification Information:**
    - Name of the head of the family: _____
    - Type of the family: _____
    - Religion: _____
    - Caste: _____
    - Address: _____

3. **Family Characteristics and Health Status of the Family Members:**

S. No.	Name of the family member	Age	Sex	Relationship with the head of the family	Education and occupation	Health (any stressor)
1.						
2.						
3.						
4.						
5.						
6.						

4. **Housing Condition:**
    - Type of house: _____
    - No. of rooms: _____
    - Ventilation: _____
    - Lighting: _____
    - Water supply: _____
    - Kitchen: _____
    - Smoke outlet: _____
    - Bath room: _____
    - Latrine: _____
    - Drainage: _____
    - Refuse disposal: _____
    - Cattle shed: _____
    - Utilization of health services: _____

5. **Socioeconomic Status:**
   - House: _____
   - Land: _____
   - Income of the family per month: _____
   - Facilities at home: _____

6. **Transport and Communication:**
   - Type of road: _____
   - Transport facilities: _____
   - Communication facilities: _____

7. **Nutritional Pattern:**
   - Food habits: _____
   _____
   - Assessment of support system: _____
   _____
   - Relationship with neighbors: _____
   - Relationship with relatives: _____

8. **Assessment of Risk Factors for Mental Health:**

S. No.	Name of family member	Present health status	Any chronic disease	Specify any stressor
1.				
2.				
3.				

- Family history of mental illness: _____
- Use of leisure: _____
- Recreational activities/relaxation activities: _____
_____
- Describe cultural practices related to health: _____
_____
- Describe religious practices/festivals: _____
_____
- Interpersonal relationship among family members: _____
_____
- Any addictions: _____
- Vital occurrence during last one year: _____
- History of past illness: _____

- **Physical handicap:** _____
- **Mental retardation:** _____
- **History of epilepsy/suicide:** _____
- **Knowledge and attitude of family about mental health and illness:** _____
_____

Summary of family visit:

Signature of Student Nurse   Signature of Supervisor

COMMUNITY MENTAL HEALTH NURSING: INDIVIDUAL CARE PLAN

An individualized care plan is a plan that is tailored to the specific needs and preferences of an individual in the community setting.

Community Mental Health Nursing: Individual Care Plan

Name	Age	Gender	Occupation/Education	Problem	Objective	Interventions	Remarks

Signature of Student Nurse

Signature of Supervisor

Name	Age	Gender	Occupation/Education	Problem	Objective	Interventions	Remarks

Signature of Student Nurse

Signature of Supervisor

Community Mental Health Nursing: Individual Care Plan

Name	Age	Gender	Occupation/Education	Problem	Objective	Interventions	Remarks

Signature of Student Nurse

Signature of Supervisor

Name	Age	Gender	Occupation/Education	Problem	Objective	Interventions	Remarks

Signature of Student Nurse

Signature of Supervisor

COMMUNITY MENTAL HEALTH NURSING: FAMILY CARE PLAN

A family care plan in the context of mental health nursing generally refers to a comprehensive and collaborative approach to supporting individuals with mental health challenges by involving their family members or significant others in the care process. The term may be used in various mental health settings, including psychiatric hospitals, outpatient clinics, or community mental health programs.

The key components of a family care plan in mental health nursing may include:
- **Assessment:** Conducting a thorough assessment of the patient's mental health status and the impact of their condition on family dynamics. This involves gathering information about family history, relationships, and support systems.
- **Collaborative goal setting:** Involving both the patient and their family members in setting treatment goals. This ensures that the care plan aligns with the needs and preferences of the individual and their support network.
- **Education:** Providing the family with information about the mental health condition, its symptoms, treatment options, and strategies for coping. Education helps families better understand the challenges their loved one is facing and fosters a supportive environment.
- **Communication:** Facilitating open and effective communication between the mental health care team, the patient, and their family. Clear communication helps in addressing concerns, providing updates on treatment progress, and involving the family in decision-making processes.
- **Crisis planning:** Developing a crisis intervention plan in collaboration with the family. This plan outlines steps to be taken in case of a mental health crisis, ensuring that the family is prepared to provide appropriate support.
- **Resource identification:** Identifying community resources and support services that can assist both the patient and their family in managing the challenges associated with mental health conditions. This may include support groups, counseling services, or respite care.
- **Follow-up and evaluation:** Regularly reviewing and evaluating the family care plan to assess its effectiveness and making adjustments as needed. Follow-up ensures that the care plan remains responsive to the evolving needs of the individual and their family.

In essence, a family care plan in mental health nursing recognizes the importance of the family unit in the well-being of individuals with mental health issues. By involving families in the care process, mental health professionals aim to create a more holistic and supportive environment that enhances the overall effectiveness of treatment and promotes long-term recovery.

Assessment of health problem	Family nursing problem	Objectives	Nursing interventions	Remarks

Community Mental Health Nursing: Family Care Plan

Assessment of health problem	Family nursing problem	Objectives	Nursing interventions	Remarks

Assessment of health problem	Family nursing problem	Objectives	Nursing interventions	Remarks

Assessment of health problem	Family nursing problem	Objectives	Nursing interventions	Remarks

DRUG BOOK

Psychiatric drugs commonly used at _____ hospital

S. No.	Generic name/brand name	Dose/Route	Class	Indication	Contraindications	Side effects	Mechanism of action	Nurses role
1.								Patient and Family Education

S. No.	Generic name/brand name	Dose/Route	Class	Indication	Contraindications	Side effects	Mechanism of action	Nurses role
2.								Patient and Family Education

S. No.	Generic name/brand name	Dose/Route	Class	Indication	Contraindications	Side effects	Mechanism of action	Nurses role
3.								Patient and Family Education

Practical Book for Mental Health Nursing–II

S. No.	Generic name/brand name	Dose/Route	Class	Indication	Contraindications	Side effects	Mechanism of action	Nurses role
4.								Patient and Family Education

S. No.	Generic name/brand name	Dose/Route	Class	Indication	Contraindications	Side effects	Mechanism of action	Nurses role
5.								Patient and Family Education

HEALTH EDUCATION

Nursing health education is concerned with the profession of nursing and the process of educating the patients, attendants regarding the care to be taken about the patients, families or communities to maintain or recover good health conditions. Health education can be given at any place like OPD, IPD.

Health Education Report

Specific objective: _____
_____
_____
_____
_____

Name of the topic: _____

Date: _____ **Time:** _____

Target population: _____

AV/AIDS Used: _____

Report:
_____
_____
_____
_____
_____
_____
_____
_____
_____
_____
_____
_____
_____

Feedback back of audience:
_____
_____

Signature of Teacher

MENTAL HEALTH CAMP

"A mental health camp is a structured and supportive program designed to promote and enhance the psychological well-being of individuals. These camps typically offer a range of therapeutic activities, counseling sessions, and educational workshops aimed at addressing various mental health issues and fostering resilience. Participants in mental health camps may include individuals experiencing stress, anxiety, depression, or other mental health challenges. The primary goal is to create a safe and inclusive environment where individuals can openly discuss their feelings, receive professional guidance, and connect with others who may share similar experiences. Mental health camps often prioritize holistic approaches to wellness, incorporating activities such as mindfulness, meditation, and expressive arts to empower participants in their journey towards improved mental health. These camps play a crucial role in reducing stigma surrounding mental health, promoting self-care, and encouraging individuals to seek help when needed."

Report on Mental Health Camp

Date: _____

Venue: _____

_____
_____
_____
_____

Objectives of Camp:

_____
_____
_____
_____
_____
_____

Report:

_____
_____
_____
_____
_____
_____
_____
_____
_____
_____
_____
_____
_____
_____

Signature of Student Nurse   **Signature of Incharge Camp**

Other Best-selling Books

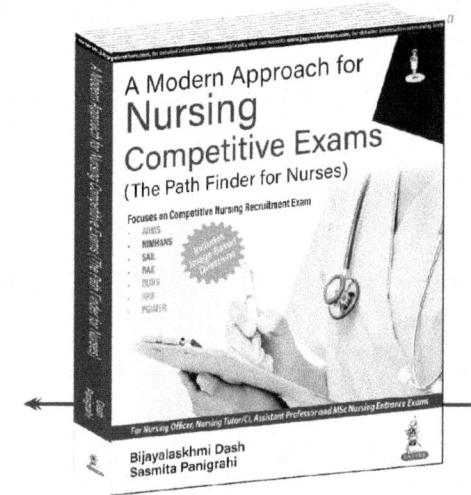

A MODERN APPROACH FOR NURSING COMPETITIVE EXAMS
(THE PATH FINDER FOR NURSES)

Bijayalaskhmi Dash, *et al.*
Single Color | Soft Cover | 1/e, 2023
8.5" x 11" | 784 Pages | 9789354659706

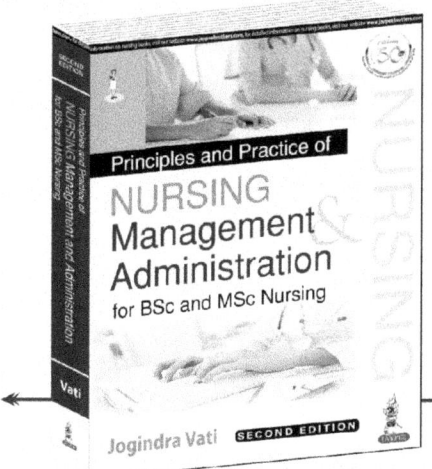

PRINCIPLES AND PRACTICE OF NURSING MANAGEMENT & ADMINISTRATION
FOR BSc AND MSc NURSING

Jogindra Vati
Single Color | Soft Cover | 2/e, 2023 (RP)
8.5" x 11" | 684 Pages | 9789390020010

JAYPEE
The Health Sciences Publisher

Please visit our website
www.jaypeebrothers.com or Scan the QR Code

EU GSPR Authorised Reprsentative
Logos Europe, 9 rue Nicolas Poussin
1700, La Rochelle, France
Phone: +33 (0) 6 67 93 73 78
E-mail: contact@logoseurope.eu

www.ingramcontent.com/pod-product-compliance
Ingram Content Group UK Ltd.
Pitfield, Milton Keynes, MK11 3LW, UK
UKHW050244150426
5217IPUK00005B/125